The Healthcare Professional's Guide to Human Research

The Healthcare Professional's Guide to Human Research

JERRY L. CRANFORD, PhD, MCD, CCC-A

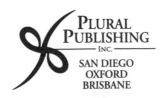

PLURAL
PUBLISHING
INC.

SAN DIEGO
OXFORD
BRISBANE

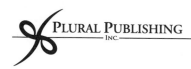

PLURAL PUBLISHING
INC.

San Diego
Oxford
Brisbane
Plural Publishing, Inc

5521 Ruffin Road
San Diego, CA 92123

e-mail: info@pluralpublishing.com
Web site: http://www.pluralpublishing.com

49 Bath Street
Abingdon, Oxfordshire OX14 1EA
United Kingdom

Copyright © by Plural Publishing, Inc. 2008

Typeset in 10½/13 Palatino by Flanagan's Publishing Services, Inc.
Printed in the United States of America by Bang Printing

For permission to use material from this text, contact us by
Telephone: (866) 758-7251
Fax: (888) 758-7255
e-mail: permissions@pluralpublishing.com

*Every attempt has been made to contact the copyright holders for material originally
printed in another source. If any have been inadvertently overlooked, the publishers will
gladly make the necessary arrangements at the first opportunity.*

Library of Congress Cataloging-in-Publication Data
Cranford, Jerry.
  The healthcare professional's guide to human research / Jerry Cranford.
      p. ; cm.
  Includes bibliographical references.
  ISBN-13: 978-1-59756-200-3 (pbk.)
  ISBN-10: 1-59756-200-9 (pbk.)
  1. Medicine--Research--Methodology. I. Title.
  [DNLM: 1. Biomedical Research--methods. W 20.5 C891h 2007]
  R850.C73 2007
  610.72--dc22

                                                    2007010322

Contents

Preface

The *Healthcare Professional's Guide to Human Research* was written as an introductory guide for physicians, nurses, and other healthcare professionals who wish to obtain a basic understanding of the essential information or tools they will need if they wish to become actively involved in research. This book assumes no prior knowledge of research design or methodology, or of statistics. The reader is introduced to the basic concepts or principles of what research is, how research projects are designed and performed, and how research data are statistically analyzed and "written up" to be reported at professional conferences or published in professional journals. The book arms the reader with enough basic knowledge to tackle required but often difficult professional reading, or to intelligently communicate with research-oriented colleagues (or consultants).

This book also will be valuable to those healthcare professionals who do not plan to be actively involved in research, but who wish to become more critical and intelligent "consumers" of the research literature. General guidelines are provided to allow the reader to critically evaluate whether a particular researcher appears to have used the appropriate research design, methodology, statistics, and so on, and to decide whether the findings and conclusions appear to have sufficient merit to allow their incorporation into the reader's own clinical practice. The advancement of the healthcare sciences, as with all fields of science, is critically dependent on the training and fostering of both competent "producers" as well as "consumers" of research.

This book was written as a basic and complete introduction to human research, with valuable information for a broad range of healthcare researchers. Although the concepts, terminology, and other relevant concepts differ markedly among the various healthcare specialty areas, the basic components and principles of the research process itself are identical. The same basic research designs and statistical tests are used regardless of whether the investigator is involved in designing improved prosthetic knee joints, developing classroom instructional protocols for a new technology, identifying psychological effects of childhood abuse, or evaluating the effectiveness of different analgesic agents in surgery. Accordingly, the content is presented in such a manner that persons with various professional backgrounds will have no difficulty understanding the basic concepts. The focus is on the principles of human research, rather than on the specialized topic areas to which these principles are applied. When examples are used to illustrate particular points, they have been selected to be applicable across all healthcare specialties and fields.

CHAPTER

1

What Is Research?
A Brief Overview

The two philosophical bases for research are *determinism* and *empiricism*. The scientist—or the clinician-investigator in the role of scientist—assumes that nothing happens by pure chance. This is the essence of determinism: All events in the real world are determined or caused by other events, or are in turn the cause of other events. Thus, the job of the scientist is to seek out and describe cause-and-effect relationships among the variables or phenomena related to a specific professional field of study.

In science, the "explanation" of natural phenomena requires detailed elucidation of the causal factors related to a particular phenomenon (Hegde, 1993; Schiavetti & Metz, 2002). In order to investigate cause-and-effect relationships, the scientist must collect data. In science, the only data that are acceptable as evidence for cause-and-effect relationships are empirical data. *Empirical data* are obtained by direct observation using the human senses, or by measurements made with calibrated instruments. Any other type of data is unacceptable to the scientist. If the data collected by one scientist are not observable and measurable, then a second scientist working at another research facility cannot attempt to verify or replicate the results of the first scientist.

In order to collect data to show evidence of cause and effect, and to allow meaningful application of the findings, the scientist must develop a formalized and systematic plan of action. This process involves a number of critical steps, summarized as follows:

1. Developing formal research questions that can be answered by the collection of appropriate empirical data.

2. Determining what kinds of data, and in what quantity, will be needed to answer the question(s).

3. Developing a strategic plan for collecting the data that will ensure that the data will, as much as possible, provide *unbiased* evidence for answering the research question(s). This step entails the development of the appropriate *research design*. Different types of research questions require different types of research design. For the data to be unbiased, the research design must incorporate certain *control conditions* to ensure that the data will be directly appropriate for answering the question(s).

4. Collecting the data. This step begins only after the first three steps have been accomplished. It is absolutely critical that the data be collected in a careful, accurate, and systematic fashion, with strict adherence to the requirements of the research design.

5. Performing statistical analysis of the collected data. The purpose of the statistical analysis, in addition to formally summarizing the major findings of the study, is to determine the likelihood that the differences or effects reflected in the data might have occurred strictly by chance. Different types of *statistical tests* are used with different types of research data. A statistical test serves as nothing more than a mathematical "neutral referee" that will provide the researcher with a probability statement of how likely it is that the results reflect a "real" finding and are not due to chance. Of course, if the researcher used the inappropriate research design, or collected the data in a sloppy fashion, the results of the statistical analysis will be both worthless and frequently misleading. Sloppy research may (and, unfortunately, often does) erroneously report findings as *statistically significant* when in fact they are not—in keeping with the adage "garbage in, garbage out!"

6. Publishing and disseminating the research findings. In this final step in the research process, the investigator's findings are made "public knowledge" so that other investigators can proceed to verify, challenge, or follow up on the research. This is the crux of the successful development of any scientific field. The researcher must present the study findings to his or her peers as one more proposed block of evidence (or "piece of the puzzle") in constructing the knowledge base of the field. The researcher's peers will then critically review the work, perhaps attempt to replicate it or expand on it, and choose to accept or reject it. To accomplish this final step, the research must be formally documented in a paper describing how the study was conducted and how the findings were derived. In writing the manuscript to be submitted for publication, the investigator must describe specifics of the research methods and findings in sufficient detail to allow other researchers to judge the importance and accuracy of the new study, as well as to replicate the study if they choose to do so.

The following chapters expand on each of these six steps, with tips on how to get the best results for the effort expended, and how to avoid common mistakes. Many newcomers to research believe that the process of doing research, with all of its varied ramifications, is extremely complex and difficult. Nothing could be further from the truth—good research need not be complex. (An especially helpful concept in this regard is that embodied in the acronym KISS—keep it simple, stupid!) Some of the best research is simple. It's true, however, that all research requires careful and accurate data collection, with constant vigilance to the procedural details required by the research design. Thus, although the researcher does not need to be a genius, it does help to be a compulsive perfectionist who can tolerate long periods of tedious data collection! Other, more attractive personality traits helpful to the professional researcher are noted throughout the book. Here, it's enough to say that Hollywood's image of the researcher as the slovenly, long-haired, eccentric, "absent-minded professor" type is pretty much a myth (there are always exceptions, of course!).

CHAPTER

2

Getting Started

Different Types of Research

Many textbooks (e.g., Hegde, 1993) on research methodology distinguish between what are considered to be two distinctively different forms of research activity—*basic* and the *applied*. In performing basic research, the investigator is thought to be pursuing answers to fundamental questions related to cause and effect, which may have no direct relevance to today's real-world clinical problems or issues. The applied researcher, on the other hand, is the one who attempts to find answers to questions that are needed to allow a solution to some immediate clinical problem.

Unfortunately, a number of common misconceptions exist regarding how these two types of research differ. Basic research, in contrast with applied research, is thought to involve a higher level of complexity and sophistication. This type of research is believed to involve pursuing solutions to more complex and difficult problems and to require the use of more complex and expensive equipment. As a result of this increased demand, it is assumed that the researcher must have a higher level of training or experience. Applied research, on the other hand, is thought to be considerably less demanding.

In truth, both basic and applied forms of research can, and commonly do, range from the simple to the complex in terms of research questions, necessary equipment, and educational or experiential background requirements for the investigator. The current pursuit of a cure for the acquired immunodeficiency syndrome (AIDS) epidemic is an excellent example of an applied clinical research problem that is quite complex in all of its different facets. The only important difference between applied and basic research is whether or not the answer to the research questions will have immediate relevance to some clinical problem. All of the basic processes of designing and conducting research are identical regardless of whether the researcher is solving an immediate clinical problem or adding one more piece of knowledge to a knowledge base that may not have any practical applications for another 20 or 30 years.

Finally, it is necessary to point out some subtle differences between the activities of the applied research scientist and the activities of the technologist (e.g., the engineer, or inventor). The engineers who take existing knowledge, whether acquired from basic or applied research, and use this information to develop better highway bridges or better mousetraps are focusing their energies on the advancement of *technology*, rather than science per se. The applied scientist uses traditional research methodology and statistics to find an answer to a practical clinical question; the technologist, in turn, uses a logical trial-and-error problem-solving approach to translate this answer into a practical and usable product. The development of new and more effective amplification systems for the hearing-impaired and of standardized test instruments for evaluating various forms of speech or language disorders constitutes an excellent example of the development of new technology in the communication disorders fields. Of course, the activities of the technologist do, on occasion, result in the discovery of unexpected new information, or in the generation of new basic or applied research questions.

Where to Begin

This chapter examines the problems related to both entering the research arena and explores how to go about selecting appropriate and manageable research questions. For the purposes of this discussion, it's assumed that the budding new researcher can take time off from busy clinical activities to conduct research studies that are independent of normal clinical practice. (A subsequent chapter addresses issues and problems related to combining research with a busy clinic schedule.) It's also assumed that the relative newcomer to research, although having considerable knowledge related to the basic science and clinical aspects of his or her professional field, knows very little about how to go about conducting either basic or applied research. Accordingly, the focus of this chapter is on pursuing simple but important research questions that will not overtax the newcomer's level of current knowledge or experience. (Readers who "get the bug" for research, perhaps with time and continued experience, can go on to tackle more complex problems.)

A number of important practical issues require careful consideration before the researcher can begin the process of developing and implementing a research project. First is the selection of a general topic area in which to conduct research. It may well be that the most successful scientist is the one who has the most fun in conducting research! To this end, it is highly recommended that the researcher select the topic area that he or she is most interested in and therefore should be most knowledgeable about and comfortable with. One of the cardinal rules of research is that the researcher must have a thorough and complete knowledge of the relevant research literature in the proposed area of investigation. It makes little sense to select a new topic area that will require a considerable amount of the new investigator's time in order to master a whole new research literature. This does not preclude a subsequent switch to a whole new field of endeavor at a later stage in the researcher's professional career. Both scientists and clinician-investigators have been known to become tired of working in the "same old field" and to switch to a new area that has piqued their interest.

The new investigator's next step is to thoroughly investigate the research literature in the chosen topic area with the goal of identifying possible gaps in the knowledge base, with some critical question or series of questions that have been neglected. Alternatively, this review of the literature may bring to light what the researcher believes to be incorrect information, on the basis of apparently inadequate or erroneous prior research. A fairly common assumption among novice researchers is that ongoing work in a particular area, coupled with considerable training and quite a bit of reading in that area, is enough to stay up to date with respect to the most recent research literature. In the communication disorders fields, however, far too many specialty journals exist to allow the typical researcher to keep abreast of all published content. The researcher, as part of the review of the literature, must perform computerized literature searches, using engines such as Medline, to identify recently published information.

It's also a good idea to identify people who are recognized as leaders and who recently have been publishing in the particular research area and to contact such persons, by letter or e-mail, requesting copies of "pre-prints" (i.e., pre-publication manuscripts) or information on any relevant research that has not yet been published. With today's professional journals, the time delay between submission of a publication manuscript and actual publication may be as long as two years. This tactic will give the researcher the greatest chance of having the most up-to-date information in the area, and perhaps prevent the embarrassment of inadvertently repeating what someone else has already done. (A subsequent section of this chapter considers the pros and cons of performing research aimed at replicating or verifying someone else's research.)

Persons in different healthcare fields, such as the graduate psychology student or the resident physician (some doctoral training programs [e.g., Au.D] in allied health and medical residency training programs do require their trainees to obtain research experience), may be expected to complete a research project; others—the teaching faculty member or hospital physical therapist, audiologist, or speech-language pathologist, for example—may decide on their own that they want to begin to do research. Whatever their impetus, both types of researchers will begin the task with no research problem or questions in mind and must go through the steps just outlined. In other cases, an individual clinician may observe something in clinical practice, perhaps related to some puzzling or unexpected finding with a patient, that triggers a question for which an answer may be of interest. At first, the question may be ill defined or vague. In order to obtain an answer to the question, the clinician must identify and define the specific topic area or areas related to the observed phenomenon and then conduct a search of the relevant healthcare literature. The answer to the question may already exist in the literature, and the clinician will not need to conduct the research project. If it does not, then the clinician may proceed to formulating an answerable research question(s) and conducting a research study. In this case, the clinician also will need to go through the steps as outlined earlier. Thus, in the real world of healthcare research, some investigators must actively seek questions to be answered, whereas others may have questions "dropped into their laps."

Seeking Help with the Research Project

Before beginning the task of formulating a final research question and developing a research design, the researcher must carefully and thoroughly check out the local situation for the necessary access to the equipment, types of research subjects, and other support facilities or people (e.g., a statistics consultant) needed to pursue the research project to a successful conclusion. One of the mistakes that many new investigators make is to assume that they must conduct the research in solo fashion. The researcher must perform a thorough personal inventory to identify the requisite skills or knowledge for performing the research. This inventory may reveal that the researcher has sufficient knowledge related to the basic science or clinical aspects of the problem area but lacks adequate knowledge or skills related to the electronic instrumentation, the research design or statistical aspects of the project, or even the skills needed to write the final publication manuscript.

Some of the best and most successful research frequently is *collaborative* research. The new researcher should seek out and attempt to recruit other professionals who would be willing to assist with the project. If, for example, the project involves complicated electronic instrumentation, and the researcher recognizes significant personal limitations in this area, a tenure-track assistant professor in the electronic engineering department at a local university may be located who is willing to work with the researcher, especially if the prospect of coauthorship on subsequent publications is offered as an incentive. In today's publish-or-perish academic and medical center environments, the offer of coauthorship frequently is as effective as, or more effective than, money as compensation for collaborating in research activities. Of course, the researcher takes some real risks when recruiting other professionals to help with a research project. As confirmed by my own research experience, some collaborators may "talk big" but fail to produce. No easy way exists to predict in advance the success or failure of any given collaborative relationship. The researcher should carefully consider the potential collaborator's background and work history. Does the person have a track record of successful and productive collaboration with other professionals? Does the level of the person's current professional activities related to teaching, research, clinical, or administrative duties appear to be excessive enough to prevent the person's realistically having sufficient time to devote to the new project?

The researcher also must carefully consider whether the project will demand more of their own time and energy than they can spare. The tendency of many new investigators (especially the highly motivated ones) is to "bite off more than they can chew" and attempt to develop complex research designs that will be far too time-consuming and demanding. Graduate students, fresh from the broad array of subject matter encountered in academic studies, are especially prone to this problem. These beginning investigators designing their first research study very often need to be convinced to "trim back" and simplify the focus of the study. The key to successful research is to develop the appropriate research design, and then carefully and accurately collect research data with *strict* adherence to the requirements of the research design. This statement sounds simple enough. As borne out by my own experience, however, it is virtually impossible for the beginning investigator to be able to accurately judge what this statement means in terms of the actual amount of time and effort required for the project. Having woefully underestimated the amount of time required, the new researcher may find that he or she cannot finish the project or, even worse, that compromises or "shortcuts" must be made to do so. It would be far better to abandon the project than to select the latter strategy and end up "polluting the scientific waters." As a rule of thumb, the beginning researcher is advised to estimate how much personal time will be needed for the project—and then multiply this number by a factor of at least 3 to be even close to the actual time that will be required! (This formula was devised from personal experience; after more than 30 years of research, I still continue to underestimate my own time requirements.) All researchers, and especially beginners, must be aware of this serious problem.

The Mentoring System in Research

An additional option may be available for some beginning researchers to lessen the pain of their induction into the world of research. As suggested earlier in this chapter, a new investigator who feels inadequate in performing research in solo fashion may consider recruiting collaborators to assist with particular facets of the project. However, even with the help of collaborators, many new investigators will still feel that their knowledge and skills in research are far too inadequate to allow them to take charge of any new project. This is especially likely to be the case with those persons whose earlier professional training included virtually no exposure to research. For readers who identify with this feeling, a less painful way to enter the research arena is suggested: Instead of enduring the difficulties and hardships inherent in developing an original project, the new researcher may consider the far less traumatic option of volunteering to be an unpaid assistant to a more experienced researcher in their own project. This *apprenticeship* or *mentoring* form of collaboration would allow the new investigator an opportunity to develop on-the-job skills in performing research under the direction of the more experienced investigator. The senior investigator, in return for this assistance, probably would be more than happy to reward the younger assistant with a coauthorship on any resulting publications.

This mentoring process is the typical means by which persons with PhD degrees in the different health science fields have traditionally received their research training. In graduate school, the budding new researcher links up with a senior clinician-investigator (professor) who becomes the researcher's major professor or advisor, and eventually the director of the student's PhD dissertation research project. The new PhD graduate may extend the mentoring process even further and elect to take a special postdoctoral fellowship or traineeship at another university or research facility to gain additional hands- on research experience under the guidance of other senior clinician-investigators.

Unfortunately, the graduates of many healthcare PhD training programs may feel that although they received excellent clinical training, they did not have an adequate opportunity to participate in a research mentoring process. However, if the new researcher is fortunate enough to be employed at a university or medical center that has experienced clinician-investigators on the staff, opportunities may develop for such mentoring relationships. The clinician who wishes to acquire research skills is encouraged to explore this possibility, if it is available. Being a "research apprentice" for a few years is a very painless and effective way to become a competent researcher. With time and experience, the clinician-investigator could graduate to doing solo research, thereby becoming an experienced senior investigator.

If the reader is on the faculty of a university that has a sabbatical program, another option would be to take a 6-month or 1-year sabbatical to spend time with an active clinician-investigator and learn how to do research. By the same token, a university faculty person with many years of solid clinical experience who elects to do a research sabbatical could, on returning to the university, be a veritable dynamo with respect to ideas for new and productive clinical research.

Formulating and Developing Viable Research Questions

After the new clinician-investigator has entered the research arena, using any of the means outlined previously, the next critical step to be mastered is to "learn how to ask" the right questions! Asking questions in science is different from asking questions in everyday life. The research question must conform to strict requirements imposed by the two philosophical tenets of science, determinism and empiricism. A question such as "Is there life after death?", although a prime consideration in the personal lives of many persons, including many scientists, is not a viable scientific question. Such questions cannot be answered with the collection of empirical data. Also, in science, the cause of an event must be some other potentially observable and measurable event. Although God may be a very viable and real entity for many people, including the scientist, "God" cannot be, for the scientist, the "cause" of anything. Science's insistence that spiritual explanations must be separated from scientific explanations should not be construed as meaning that scientists deny the existence of God. In their everyday work, scientists must restrict themselves to pursuing questions that can be answered only with empirical data.

In science, the *development* or *formulation* of a research question has a very special meaning that must be distinguished from the layman's concept of the simple "asking" of a question. To answer the question, the scientist must know exactly what is being asked. The layperson may, when hearing the question, ask "What do you mean by such-and-such?" The scientist, by contrast, must operationally define the concepts or terms that are used in the research question. For beginning researchers, it's a good idea to precede their first research project by preparing a written research proposal that begins with a detailed *statement* and *explanation* of the research question or questions to be investigated. This document consists of a statement of the research question(s) followed by a series of *operational definitions* of the terms or concepts used in the question(s). The operational definitions serve to define what is meant by the terms or concepts, plus define exactly what kind of data will be needed to answer the question(s). The following examples are presented to clarify this process.

Example 2–1: Initial wording of the research question: "Does administration of a particular clinical treatment program reduce the severity of dysfluency (i.e., stuttering) in children?"

In order to design a research study to answer this question, the investigator must provide operational definitions for the key terms of *severity*, *dysfluency*, and *children*, as well as *particular clinical treatment program*. Each of these concepts, without further elaboration or "tighter" definition, is quite broad and rather "fuzzy" with respect to its exact meaning. In operationally defining these concepts, the researcher must specify exactly what kinds of empirical data will be used to define the concept. The operational definition of dysfluency would include the specific type or category of dysfluency (e.g., x or y) as determined by scores achieved on one particular standardized evaluation measure (e.g., the "XYZ-Revised test, version 2") of dysfluency. Changes in scores before and after the administration of the treatment program will constitute the data that will reflect the change in severity of stuttering. In this study, changes in severity of dysfluency will be operationally defined as "changes in scores on the XYZ-Revised, version 2 test." Likewise, *children* may be operationally defined as "males from middle class family backgrounds between the ages of 12 and 15 years." Thus, the scientist typically uses very restricted definitions for the terms or concepts used in the research question. Another scientist may operationally define stuttering in a completely different manner, but this investigator too would have to restrict the definitions to involving only measurable and publicly verifiable data. In designing the actual research project, the researcher must, of course, spell out what the researcher means or intends to do, with respect to a number of other aspects of the research question, such as the following: "What specific treatment protocol will be administered, and for how long?" "How many children will be tested?" This study would involve an experimental design (or, possibly, a prospective outcomes design) in which a specific cause-and-effect relationship—for example, whether a particular clinical treatment routine "causes" the "effect" of reduced severity levels of dysfluency in children—is investigated. The researcher also must therefore describe in detail the *control* methods that he or she will use to ensure that any observed changes in severity of dysfluency are indeed due to the administration of the treatment and not to some other *uncontrolled* variable(s).

Example 2–2: Initial wording of the research question: "Does prosthetic knee joint A produce better long-term outcomes than prosthetic device B?"

Across all healthcare specialty fields, outcomes research has, in recent years, emerged as a major player in the research arena. With this particular research question, the investigator must provide a detailed operational definition of what kind of data will be collected and how those data will be used to define what constitutes a *better* outcome. The researcher also must define what is meant by *long-term*. In developing the research design, the investigator also must spell out how many patients will be studied, and what control procedures (e.g., matching the two groups with respect to age, sex, physical characteristics, health status, physical activity levels—whether sedentary office worker or telephone line worker) will be used to ensure that any differences found in the outcomes data will reflect which prosthetic device was implanted and not some incidental difference between the two patient groups.

In some textbooks on research methods, it is specified that, rather than asking research questions, the investigator must pose a *hypothesis* to be *tested* in the research study. The hypothesis, in this sense, is a formal prediction of the outcome of the study. Thus, a research question such as "Does drug X improve memory functions in children with epilepsy?" could be restated in a hypothesis format as follows: "Drug X produces significant improvements in the memory functions of children with epilepsy." Now, instead of obtaining a yes-or-no answer to a research question, the researcher gathers data that would provide evidence that supports the predicted outcome of the study, or that fails to support or even contradicts the hypothesis.

In some formal research textbooks, it may further be specified that, in order to be truly scientific, the predicted outcome must be phrased in the form of a *null hypothesis* The null hypothesis, as the term indicates, predicts a "null" or nonsignificant outcome of the research study. In this format, the original question would be restated as follows: "Drug X produces no significant changes in the memory functions of children with epilepsy." It is argued that, because researchers are supposed to be totally unbiased with respect to the outcomes of their research, the use of the null hypothesis somehow demonstrates to the world the researcher's intent to be unbiased in his or her work. The scientist's null hypothesis is analogous to the "innocent until proven guilty" concept in law. A later chapter on statistics describes how the concept of the null hypothesis has been incorporated into the process of interpreting the outcome of inferential statistical testing.

Finally, a brief discussion of some issues related to the so-called *quality* or *scientific merit* of particular research questions is in order. Although some research questions may be considered to be more important than others, why they are more important may at times be more closely tied to the collective bias (the prevailing zeitgeist) of the scientific community than to actual scientific truth. At any given time, and in all fields of science, some topics are considered to be "hot," whereas others are currently less interesting or "exciting." The new researcher would be wise to take this factor into account when selecting a topic for his or her first research project. Given a choice between what the researcher believes are two equally important questions, it may be prudent to select the one that the professional community would be more interested in seeing investigated. In a later chapter, some common pitfalls in healthcare research related to the human nature of the individual scientist, and to the collective biases of the scientific community, are considered.

3

Developing a Plan of Action

This chapter looks at the process of designing the research study. The previous chapter described the steps involved in developing and formulating the research question or questions. The nature of the research question will dictate the type of data that must be collected to answer the question. The *research design* will, in turn, dictate the specific manner in which the data must be collected in order to ensure the most accurate answer to the research question(s).

Different research questions require different types of research designs. As noted in Chapter 1, the primary goal in all fields of science is to identify and describe, in detail, the specific cause-and-effect relationships of all of the natural phenomena that are unique to a particular field. In the behavioral sciences, it is essential to distinguish between *nonexperimental* and *experimental* research designs. The nature of the research question will dictate which type of design must be used in any given research project. The two types of designs differ in how effective they are with respect to establishing evidence for cause and effect. The experimental design provides *direct* evidence for cause and effect by allowing the researcher to actively manipulate possible causal variables and to determine which ones produce the predicted effects. With nonexperimental designs, the potential causes are not available for the researcher to actively manipulate. The researcher must use statistical correlation techniques to provide *indirect* anecdotal evidence of cause-and-effect relationships. In this book, the term *research* is used in the generic sense to refer to both nonexperimental and experimental designs. Whenever the research design is experimental in nature, however, the study is referred to as an experiment or as involving an experimental design.

Five basic types of nonexperimental and experimental designs commonly are used in behavioral research. A brief description of each type is presented next.

Brief Overview of Different Research Designs

In the healthcare fields, the nonexperimental *case study designs* involve detailed description of the unique characteristics or features of individuals or groups of persons with specific forms of a specific medical or health-related disorder. Research of this type attempts to define what is typical with respect to a given condition. Such descriptive studies are needed as precursors to later research designs that attempt to identify causal factors or develop possible treatments. Shortly after discovery of the disease, the flurry of descriptive studies in patients with acquired immunodeficiency syndrome (AIDS) illustrates this point quite well. In the speech and hearing sciences, and in other behavioral fields (e.g., psychology, physical therapy), this type of design also can refer to descriptions of the *normal* expected behaviors of specific groups of people. Studies of the expected developmental milestones of language or motor skills of children at different ages are examples of such *normative* study designs.

A second commonly used nonexperimental design, which also is descriptive, involves detailed comparison of persons with a given health-related disorder with persons who do not have the disorder. This design frequently is referred to as the *standard group comparison design*. This type of research goes one very critical step beyond that of the case study design by attempting to specify and measure exactly how a *clinical* group (of persons with the disorder, for example) differs from a *nonclinical* or standard group (of persons without the disorder). The two groups need to be matched with respect to all critical variables (e.g., age, sex, socioeconomic status) except for the presence or absence of the disorder.

Although the case study or normative designs and the standard group comparison designs are purely descriptive in nature and provide no direct or even indirect evidence of cause-and-effect relationships, a third form of nonexperimental design, formally labeled the *ex post facto design*, frequently is used to answer questions regarding the original cause or causes of current medical conditions. In the healthcare sciences, these designs frequently are referred to as *historical* or *retrospective* studies. The possibility of some form of causal link between chronic otitis media (i.e., middle ear infections or another pathologic condition) in young children and subsequent developmental language problems was determined with this type of design. *Medical chart studies* also are a common example of this type of design. In contrast with the first two nonexperimental designs described previously, ex post facto designs can provide indirect evidence of possible cause-and-effect relationships among variables.

A fourth type of nonexperimental design has, in recent years, become very popular in all healthcare professions, including that of communication disorders. It is a direct response to the recent increased insistence by insurance agencies and third party providers that specific treatment procedures must be shown, through research studies or other means, to be effective in order to qualify for reimbursement. These types of designs, frequently referred to as *outcomes research designs* (several distinct varieties of these designs exist, as described later on), are similar in many ways to the ex post facto design except that they typically are *prospective* rather than retrospective. Rather than "looking backwards" for the cause of some current phenomenon, the researcher "looks forward" to determine the effects (outcome) of some current causal variable (e.g., a treatment procedure for a specific form of language disorder or disease condition).

Although normative and standard group comparison designs are valuable techniques for obtaining detailed descriptive data related to the unique characteristics of individuals with specific disorders, they provide no evidence for cause and effect. By contrast, although ex post facto and outcomes research designs, when carefully executed, can provide the researcher with indirect evidence or suggestions as to possible causal factors, only the *experimental design* has the potential to provide direct unequivocal evidence of cause and effect. The experiment actually introduces possible *causal variables* (such as treatments) and determines whether or not the predicted *effect* actually occurs. In the behavioral disorders fields, and especially speech-language pathology, researchers distinguish between two basic forms of experimental design, referred to as *between-group* and *single-subject* designs (described in detail later in the chapter).

These five basic types of research designs are the ones most commonly used in healthcare research in which behavioral or functional changes in patients are being investigated (e.g., medical treatments, physical therapies, language disorders). Specific healthcare studies, however, may and frequently do use a combination of more than one of the designs to tackle specific research questions. These are referred to as mixed or *hybrid* research designs.

The following sections provide in-depth descriptions of the unique characteristics of each of the different types of designs, describe how each design typically is set up and executed, and finally considers the strengths and weaknesses of each design with respect to providing evidence of cause-and-effect relationships.

Normative or Case Study Designs

In the development of any new field of investigation, the first order of business for the scientist is to develop complete, accurate, and thorough descriptions of the different natural phenomena that the specific field or discipline will be involved in studying. In science, obtaining detailed *description* and *measurement* of natural phenomena is a critical and necessary precursor to "explaining" natural phenomena—that is, to identifying cause-and-effect relationships. The normative or case study designs, therefore, provide the basic, "bread-and-butter" information needed for development of the behavioral healthcare disorders fields (Hegde, 1993). These types of studies are designed to provide detailed descriptions of the unique characteristics or features of persons with specific or unusual forms of healthcare problems. They also frequently are designed to determine what is the expected "normal" function or characteristic of specific categories of patients or other populations. Although these types of studies are not primarily concerned with identifying possible causative factors related to specific medical conditions or behavioral functions, they frequently provide valuable clues regarding causation. In speech-language pathology, for example, considerable normative research has been performed to identify and describe the expected normal speech and language behaviors of children at different ages. Having knowledge of the normal language behavior of children allows the speech-language pathologist to determine whether the language behavior of a specific child is normal or abnormal for age and also may provide clues to what may be the cause of the child's problem.

In performing normative or case study research, the researcher needs to maintain focus on what data already have been published related to the specific topic. These types of studies typically are not done in isolation but are aimed at adding new information to an already existing data pool. Of course, case studies occasionally may be involved with describing what the researcher believes is the first or original case of its type, or at least one that is extremely rare. A major goal of these basic types of descriptive studies should be, however, to confirm, refute, or expand on similar descriptive data that have been previously published by other investigators. In writing the publication manuscript, the researcher must devote considerable time and effort to describing how his or her findings compare with those of earlier investigations. If, over the span of several years, several investigators report (and compare) findings on a series of instances of the same extremely rare case, the cumulative effect will be a more complete understanding of a specific rare disease entity.

Likewise, using a *comparative approach* in collecting normative data on groups of subjects also can expand current understanding of the basic phenomena of a particular field. For example, in a study conducted in Boston, Massachusetts, of the typical or expected age-related language or speech characteristics of children, the researcher may find that the data differ from those previously published by an investigator who conducted a similar study with children living in Montgomery, Alabama. The cumulative effect of these two studies taken together would be to further expand the field's knowledge of the typical age-related speech-language behaviors of children, and also to add valuable new information related to the influences of differences related to regional dialect.

Standard Group Comparison Designs

The standard group comparison design, like the normative or case study design, is aimed at developing a detailed description or understanding of the specific characteristics of certain types of patients. The standard group comparison design, however, includes a very critical and important element of control that is absent in the former type of design. These studies involve a detailed comparison of a *clinical* group with a nonclinical or *standard* group. The clinical group consists of a group of persons who exhibit the specific form of healthcare disorder that the clinician-investigator is interested in describing and measuring. The standard group consists of persons who are matched to those in the clinical group with respect to other critical variables (age, sex, educational or socioeconomic background, and so on) except that they do not exhibit the specific disorder. This allows the researcher to describe *how* and *in exactly what ways* persons who have the condition differ from those who do not.

Standard group comparison studies typically use one of two basic approaches in comparing the clinical and the standard groups. With the first approach, the researcher further investigates differences between the two groups on the same criterion variable that separated the groups in the first place. For example, if the criterion variable is the presence of speech and language problems (e.g., aphasia) in patients who have experienced a stroke, the researcher would further describe the specific manner in which the speech and language behaviors or skills of aphasic patients differs from persons who have not had a stroke. This type of study would provide a more detailed and complete description of exactly how the language and speech behaviors of aphasic stroke patients differs from that of persons who do not exhibit signs of aphasia. For this study to be successful, however, the two groups of research subjects would need to be matched in terms of age, sex, education level, and native language and dialect, plus any other *premorbid characteristics* (i.e., characteristics that were present in the stroke patient group before the occurrence of the stroke) that might normally have differentiated the speech and language characteristics of the two groups of subjects.

The second approach used in standard group comparison research is to investigate differences between the two groups on variables that are different from the criterion variable that initially was used to separate the two groups. Whereas the first approach is purely descriptive in nature, these latter studies usually are focused on providing anecdotal evidence as to the possible cause(s) of the specific medical condition. The researcher may be interested in testing a "hunch" or a hypothesis that he or she has developed regarding the cause of the specific condition. For example, after conducting a descriptive study of the specific speech and language differences between aphasic and nonaphasic stroke patients, the researcher may develop the idea that the difficulty that aphasic stroke patients have in understanding spoken language may be the result of a more basic problem related to short-term memory, rather than a problem with language function per se. At the time that they hear the last part of the sentence, such patients may not be able to remember what was said at the beginning of the sentence. In this case, the researcher would design a new study to determine if aphasic stroke patients have poorer short-term memory capacities than do nonaphasic patients. The new study might approach this problem by using stimuli from other sensory modalities, such as vision or somatosensory (touch), to determine if the problem is specific to the auditory (hearing) modality or is modality independent.

Unfortunately, studies that use the standard group comparison design frequently are described in the professional literature as "experiments," with the clinical and standard groups are referred to as the "experimental" and "control" groups, respectively. The use of these terms may mislead some readers into believing that the study obtained stronger evidence of cause and effect than is actually the case. The standard group comparison design provides descriptive data only, and observed differences between the clinical and standard groups should never be interpreted as providing any more than anecdotal clues or suggestions as to what may be the actual cause(s) of the condition.

Ex Post Facto Designs

As the term indicates, *ex post facto designs* seek to obtain "after the fact" or retrospective evidence of the cause or causes of some current phenomenon. In many instances, the original cause of the current healthcare disorder is something that happened in the past and consequently is no longer available for the researcher to study. In searching for these possible causes, the researcher must delve into the patient's history to obtain evidence of what the original predisposing or causal factors might have been.

Because of the fact that in ex post facto research, the potential "causes" are separated from the potential "effects" by significant periods of time, the researcher cannot hope to manipulate both types of variables in the same research project. However, this fact should not prevent the researcher from implementing certain *control procedures* to increase the likelihood that the indirect evidence obtained for the hypothesized cause-and-effect relationship is as accurate as possible. Various control procedures can be used with retrospective research. Examples of these procedures are discussed next.

In performing a retrospective study to identify possible historical causes of a specific communication disorder, the researcher needs to simultaneously study two groups of patients. The first group, the *clinical group*, is a group of patients who exhibit the condition. The second group, the *nonclinical group*, is a group of subjects who are similar to the subjects in the clinical group in all respects except that they are free of the specific medical condition. The critical word here is *similar*! Ideally, the clinical and the nonclinical groups should be essentially clones of each other except for the presence or absence of the specific disorder. Because that is not possible, the researcher must do the next best thing and try to match the two groups on all critical variables that may possibly influence whether or not the medical disorder occurs in a particular patient.

An example of a controlled ex post facto study can be cited from the field of speech-language pathology. Many years ago, early researchers in the field (Johnson, 1955; Johnson et al., 1959) began an ex post facto study to investigate the possible cause for dysfluency (stuttering) in children. Johnson and his associates conducted extensive and detailed interviews with the parents of both dysfluent children (clinical group) and nondysfluent (nonclinical group) children in an attempt to identify common factors or events that might have distinguished the two groups at the time that stuttering first began. These researchers used a structured questionnaire format to ensure that the same questions were asked of both groups of parents. The researchers found that both groups of children did, in fact, exhibit "normal" dysfluent productions (stuttering) in their speech that reflected the fact that they had not yet mastered the speech system. However, whereas the parents of the nonstuttering children apparently recognized that this dysfluent behavior reflected a normal learning process, the parents of the stuttering children reported that they became "concerned" that the child had a problem that needed professional attention. From this evidence, Johnson's team theorized that one possible cause of stuttering may involve the negative consequences related to the parents' somehow transferring their anxiety to the child. The children now became anxious and concerned about their own speech, thereby triggering the development of stuttering. Subsequent research on the causes of stuttering in children have found that this common disorder comes in many different varieties and has multiple causative factors, only one of which is the parental anxiety factor demonstrated in Johnson's research studies.

In the foregoing example, and with ex post facto research in general, the researcher is forced to rely on anecdotal or historical data to provide evidence for identifying the possible cause(s) of some current medical or healthcare condition. Such data are fraught with a multitude of possible flaws that can easily invalidate their usefulness for these purposes. Medical chart entries may or not have been entered accurately, or may not have been entered at all in many cases. Over the span of many years, the criteria for what data are entered, how accurately or completely they are entered, and so on, all change in an uncontrolled fashion. The entries also are made by a multitude of different nurses, physicians, and healthcare specialists whose biases, judgments, and even clarity of handwritten notations can vary widely. Likewise, interviews conducted with individual patients, or the patient's family members, are fraught with uncontrolled and unpredictable errors related to memory and personal bias. Despite these problems, however, the retrospective investigative approach continues to be the only viable means of seeking evidence related to the historical cause(s) of many current healthcare disorders.

Outcomes Research Designs

In recent years, *outcomes research* has rapidly gained popularity in all of the healthcare fields, including that of audiology and speech-language pathology. Although ex post facto and outcomes research are similar in many ways, they differ in one very significant fashion. With the retrospective design, the researcher has knowledge of the *effect* (e.g., the current phenomenon or communication disorder) and must search for evidence of unknown *causal* factors that may have been operative in the past. With outcomes research, in marked contrast, the researcher begins the investigation with knowledge of the potential historical causal factor(s) and then proceeds to search for future unknown effects (*outcomes*).

The same control procedures that are required for retrospective or ex post facto studies also are needed for these prospective designs. These studies should be set up to compare the outcomes of a given treatment (or procedure) in a clinical group of subjects with the outcomes found with another type of treatment or procedure (or no treatment) in a nonclinical group. In performing such studies, it is critical that the researchers limit their study to a comparison of two groups of patients who are matched on all known incidental or extraneous variables that may make a difference in how the patient adjusts or responds to the different treatments.

Outcomes research can be either preplanned or performed in a post hoc fashion. The post hoc variety has been, until recently, the most commonly used type of outcomes research. The recent medical literature refers to these types of projects as *retrospective outcomes research*. In these studies, the researcher develops the outcomes project by artificially forming two matched groups of subjects. One group, sometimes referred to as the *clinical* group, is randomly drawn from a larger pool of patients who had earlier received a specific treatment (or drug, medical device, or other treatment). A second group of patients (frequently referred to as the *nonclinical* group) is also drawn from a nonmedical group or a patient group that did not specifically receive the treatment (or drug, device, or other). It is very important that both clinical and nonclinical groups be matched with each other as closely as possible on all physiological or medical history characteristics that may have made a difference in how the patients responded to the treatments, or how they theoretically would have responded if given the treatment or drug.

Both subject groups are brought back to the clinical facility and administered a battery of tests (e.g., behavioral, functional/physiological, blood assays, genetic profiles) to determine whether any differences can be identified that can be causally linked to having received the medical procedure (treatment, device, or drug) Thus, the retrospective outcomes design involves measurement of current "effects" that may constitute a clinical outcome for some medical procedure administered in the past. These studies suffer from many of the same interpretation problems or limitations as with the traditional ex post facto or historical designs as described. Neither the clinical or nonclinical patients were intended to be part of a subsequent research study, and as a consequence, specific procedural details may not have been recorded or may have varied widely from patient to patient. As a result, the individual members of the different research groups formed in this manner may differ with respect to critical (and possibly unknown) variables that may contaminate and thus severely limit interpretation of the later outcomes data.

In recent years, a *controlled* form of outcomes research has become increasingly popular in many healthcare fields. The term *prospective outcomes research* has been coined for this variety of project. In these studies, the researcher selects two groups of patients who have a specific medical condition that requires treatment. It is critical that the two groups of patients be matched on *all known physiological* or *behavioral/functional characteristics* in addition to the presence of the specific disorder. Thus, once again, two groups of patients that are virtually clones of each other would work best, but now the "cloning" also should include the medical condition that is the target of the investigation. Because cloning is not possible, the subjects must be randomly assigned to one or the other group or matched on critical variables. The researcher then begins administering the experimental treatment (or drug) to one group and an alternative treatment (the current standard treatment, or even no treatment (i.e., a *placebo* in the form of a sham treatment or a bogus drug) to the other group. Information as to group membership (i.e., who gets the drug or treatment versus who does not) is kept secret from the individual patients, as well as from those research staff members who do not need to know. The use of such *blinded* research protocols prevents any personal bias of the subjects or staff from contaminating the study outcome.

After a period of several days, weeks, or months (however long the study needs to be), the researcher examines the research subjects to determine specific differences with respect to the outcomes. In some studies, the outcomes data are continually measured at regular intervals during the course of the investigation. If evidence begins to appear that strongly suggests that the drug or treatment is working, and the severity of the medical condition warrants it, the researchers may elect to "break protocol" and stop the study short of its original planned termination date. This would allow both groups to now get what appears to be a more beneficial treatment protocol. Prospective outcomes studies are thus designed and developed from the very outset using rigorous research control procedures. When carefully performed, these studies can approach the scientific rigor of the experimental group designs (described later in this chapter) with respect to their ability to obtain direct evidence for cause and effect. The greatest hazard to the success of these studies, however, is the inordinately long periods of time that typically intervene between the administration of possible causal variables (e.g., treatments) and the subsequent measurement of the effects (outcomes). With longer intervening time periods, the chance increases that incidental variables (e.g., lifestyle changes, changes in health status) may occur that will "override" and change the patient's final response to the original treatment. In conducting such long-term outcomes research, the investigators must be vigilant to the possible occurrence of such *confounding variables*.

In recent years, marked increases in healthcare costs have spurred the insurance companies and other third party providers to become increasingly insistent on seeing validated proof that specific treatments are truly effective. This has provided a major incentive for the rapid growth of outcomes research in all healthcare fields. Thus, despite the many difficulties involved in conducting effective outcomes research, such projects are springing up at medical centers all over the country. The National Institutes of Health (NIH) has started channeling larger amounts of money into these projects; in many instances, the projects involve coordinated studies in which data are collected from patients at multiple institutions. These types of studies also are helping to break down the traditional barrier to outcomes research related to the time factor. The NIH is becoming increasingly willing to allow such studies to continue for longer and longer periods.

An important point is that the terminology used to describe or label the different forms of retrospective and prospective outcomes research may differ according to the purpose or intent of a specific research study. Because many retrospective outcomes studies use information from the patient's documented history (i.e., medical chart), they sometimes are referred to as *medical chart studies*. Those prospective outcomes studies that focus on investigating the effectiveness of different treatment procedures frequently are labeled *treatment efficacy studies*, and studies that investigate the effectiveness of some type of drug or medical device are referred to as *clinical trials research*.

More on Retrospective and Prospective Research Designs

To further illustrate both the unique strengths and the inherent weaknesses of *retrospective* and *prospective* research approaches, the use of these two designs to investigate a special problem in the speech-language pathology field is described next. This relates to the effects of otitis media (i.e., middle ear pathology or infections) in infants and young children on later speech and language development.

A considerable amount of animal research strongly suggests that depriving the young animal of normal sensory input (either visual or auditory) impedes the normal physiological development of those areas of the nervous system involved in processing such information (Bach-Y-Rita, 1990; Bishop, 1982; Cotman, 1985). Some animal research indicates the existence of certain critical periods in the development of the brain during which, if normal sensory input is not available, the neural structures related to that specific sensory modality will fail to develop in a normal fashion. These effects are thought by some scientists to be permanent and irreversible. Many professionals in the communication science fields are concerned that the lack of normal auditory sensory input that results from chronic otitis media in young children may have a similar deleterious effect on the development of the portions of the nervous system involved in hearing and language functions (Roberts, Wallace, & Henderson, 1997).

All of the clinical research in this area has involved the use of either retrospective or prospective research approaches. When using the *retrospective* or historical approach, the investigators typically formed matched groups of children who were similar in all critical variables (e.g., age, socioeconomic status, ethnic or racial background), except that one group (i.e., the clinical group) had documented evidence of delayed or impaired language-processing abilities, whereas the other group (the nonclinical group) exhibited normal language function. The medical histories of the two groups of children were then searched to determine whether the children in the language-impaired group had exhibited a significantly higher incidence of chronic otitis media during the first year or two of life. Many of these studies have provided evidence that among children who later exhibit language problems, the incidence of early otitis media is significantly greater than among children who are free of this early childhood disease.

Investigations that used the *prospective* approach, by contrast, formed groups of older children who were matched on all critical variables except for the incidence of early otitis media. Children in the clinical group had a history of early otitis media, whereas those in the nonclinical group did not. The investigators then administered language tests to determine whether children who had a history of early otitis media would perform more poorly than children who had been free of otitis media. Many of these prospective studies have confirmed the results of their retrospective counterparts in finding a significant correlation between the occurrence of early otitis media and later language problems. In recent years, a few clinician-investigators have extended such prospective studies to involve the longitudinal assessment of children beginning at very young ages with the tests repeated at regular intervals over periods of several months or years. These projects are designed to evaluate whether early otitis media is somehow associated with delays in the emergence of certain language skills and also whether the affected children may later "catch up" with their normal peers.

As noted, both retrospective and prospective research designs have inherent limitations and can never provide any better than indirect or anecdotal evidence of cause-and-effect relationships. The finding of a significant correlation between early otitis media and later language impairment does not, therefore, prove the existence of a causal relationship between the two conditions. Many researchers have criticized this type of research on the basis of the manner in which the different groups of children were originally matched. A number of other factors or variables are known to influence both the incidence of otitis media and levels of language function in children. One critical variable relates to socioeconomic status. Children from families of lower socioeconomic status may, because of the lower educational level of the parents, experience impoverished language stimulation and, because of a less healthy living environment and poorer diet, also experience a higher incidence of associated otitis media. Thus, unless the clinical and nonclinical groups of children are carefully matched with respect to socioeconomic status, the researcher will not be able to determine whether the later language problems were due to lack of early language stimulation or lack of normal auditory stimulation as a result of the hearing loss associated with the otitis media.

Also, young children who suffer from recurrent bouts of otitis media frequently are sick and therefore less attentive to environmental sounds, and also miss more days of school, which in turn deprives them of the normal intellectual stimulation associated with school activities. Therefore, in addition to hearing loss, a multitude of other potential causal factors may be associated with the presence of early otitis media. Thus, although retrospective or prospective correlation designs are the only viable means available for investigating possible causal relationships between early otitis media and impaired language development in children, they can never provide a definitive answer to the question of what is the specific cause(s) of the subsequent language problem.

Experimental Research Designs

The only way in which a researcher can obtain direct evidence for cause-and-effect relationships in natural phenomena is to actively manipulate a possible causal variable and see if the predicted effect actually occurs. With both ex post facto and outcomes research designs, the inordinate amount of time that separates the "cause" from the "effect" variables makes it impossible or extremely difficult for a researcher to be able to effectively and accurately manipulate and measure both variables in a single research project. With ex post facto designs, the potential causative variables are ones that occurred in the past and are no longer available to be actively manipulated by the researcher. Likewise, with outcomes research designs, the potential causes and effects may be separated by months, years, or even decades. Only the most patient, persistent, and compulsive of researchers would be able to keep a project going that long!

A point warranting emphasis is that the use of nonexperimental designs is in no way a "weaker" or "less scientific" means of doing research. Many of the important questions that healthcare disorders specialists must investigate cannot be answered with experimental designs. The nature of the phenomena being investigated will dictate the type of research design that must be used. The indirect evidence for cause and effect that is provided by nonexperimental research may be the best evidence that can be obtained. The problem that these designs pose is the fact that, without being able to manipulate and test the effects of various possible causative variables, the researcher can never be sure that the variable he or she thinks was the cause actually *is* the cause. Another unknown variable may have been present that is the real cause. With an experiment, the researcher can actively *test* each of a number of potential causative variables and thereby determine which one(s) actually cause the predicted effects.

Researchers typically prefer to use the terms *independent variable* and *dependent variable*, rather than cause and effect, when describing experimental designs. The independent variable is actively manipulated by the researcher, and the effects of this manipulation are determined by measuring changes in a specific dependent variable. The most common way in which independent variables are manipulated is to form groups of *experimental* and *control* subjects. The experimental group receives a specific treatment, whereas the control group receives a different treatment or, in some studies, no treatment at all. In conducting experimental studies, the researcher must implement a number of critical *control procedures*. In all experiments, it is important that the two groups of subjects be as similar as possible with respect to all known variables except for the independent (manipulated) variable. In some studies, it also is important that, between the time that the independent variable is administered (or, in some control groups, not administered) and the time at which effects on the dependent variable are measured, subjects in the experimental and control groups be treated in a similar fashion.

It is mandatory that subjects in the experimental and control groups be matched on as many critical variables as possible that potentially may differentially affect how they will respond to the independent variable. The goal of the experiment is to *isolate* the effects of the independent variable on the dependent variable. If the experimental and the control subjects are found to differ on the dependent measure, the researcher will want to know that this effect is not due to some difference between the subjects in the two groups with respect to some other, uncontrolled or *extraneous variable*. An extraneous variable is any difference between the experimental and control groups that potentially may differentially affect how the subjects will respond to the independent variable.

The definition of what constitutes a critical extraneous variable will differ from experiment to experiment. In designing the study, the researcher must carefully consider and make a list of all those specific subject characteristics which, if allowed to differ between the experimental and control groups, might make a difference in how subjects respond on the dependent measure. Differences related to age, sex, medical history, socioeconomic or educational factors, and so on are common extraneous variables that must be controlled for in many healthcare disorders research projects.

In conducting experimental research, either of two different methods commonly are used to control for extraneous differences between experimental and control groups. One procedure involves *random assignment* of subjects to the experimental and control groups. With this method, the researcher selects an initial group of, say, 100 subjects, and then uses some unbiased or "neutral" means of randomly assigning individual subjects to form two equivalent groups of 50 subjects. A simple flip of the coin may be used for this purpose, or the researcher can consult a special table of random numbers (which can be found in most statistics textbooks). Subjects with "heads" or "even numbers" could be assigned to the experimental group, and those with "tails" or "odd numbers" would be assigned to the control group. The advantage of using such random procedures for subject assignment is that, theoretically, all extraneous variables, known as well as unknown, should be matched between the two groups.

The use of random procedures usually works quite well for matching subject groups, but only if the number of subjects is large. The larger the number of subjects, the better the method works. However, if the research study involves fewer than 50 subjects, a substantial risk exists for the presence of chance differences between the two groups in some critical extraneous variable. It is strongly recommended that, with smaller groups of subjects, the researcher match the experimental and control groups with respect to all known critical variables. This can be achieved in one of two ways. The first involves matching subject to subject. This method is variously referred to as *yoked-pair* or simply *paired-subject* matching. The researcher selects two subjects at a time who are closely matched on all critical variables and then randomly assigns one of the subjects to the experimental group and one to the control group. The researcher then selects a second pair of closely matched subjects and again randomly assigns them to the two groups. The second method of matching involves forming two groups that are statistically matched with regard to known critical variables. Thus, with this procedure, the researcher will form groups in which the averages and degrees of intersubject variation for each of the critical extraneous variables are the same for the experimental and the control groups. Thus, for example, if age and audiometric threshold levels are considered to be critical variables, the two groups would have the same mean age and sensory hearing levels—and the within-group variances (e.g., standard deviations, discussed in a later chapter) would be equivalent for each of these measures. Although the random assignment of subjects to experimental and control groups should, if the subject groups are large enough, ensure that the groups will be matched on unknown as well as known extraneous variables, with use of matching procedures the groups may not be matched with respect to unknown variables. Thus, the researcher must take extra care when using matching procedures to make sure that all known extraneous variables have been controlled for.

Between-Group versus Single-Subject Experimental Designs

The goal of the experimental design is to investigate the effects of specific independent variables on specific dependent variables. This provides direct evidence for the presence of hypothesized cause-and-effect relationships. Researchers commonly refer to this process as demonstrating *experimental control*—showing that when the independent variable is present (e.g., when the treatment is administered), a specific effect or change occurs in the dependent variable, and when the variable is absent, no change or effect is observed. In *between-group experimental designs*, this experimental control is demonstrated by the observed differences between the experimental and the control groups in the dependent measure. In psychology and speech-language pathology, a different form of experimental design has been developed in which the demonstration of experimental control is based on effects or changes observed within the individual patient, rather than between different subjects.

This type of design is referred to as the *single-subject experimental design* (Kearns, 1986; McReynolds & Kearns, 1983, 1986).

The single-subject experimental design has its historical origins in experimental psychology. During the 1950s, B. F. Skinner, an experimental psychologist at Harvard University, became disillusioned with the methods that psychologists were using to investigate the learning capabilities of animals. The traditional method of performing learning studies involved training large numbers of animals on discrimination tasks and then using the averaged data from all the animals as the bases for developing theories related to the behavioral mechanisms involved in animal learning. Such studies used the between-group experimental strategy, in which performances of groups of experimental animals were compared to groups of control animals. Skinner argued that such group data cannot accurately portray how the individual animal learns. Skinner developed a whole new approach to animal research in which he and his students placed the focus on studying the behaviors of individual animals, rather than of groups of animals.

In speech-language pathology, the single-subject design is well suited to evaluating the effectiveness of specific treatment regimens (McReynolds & Kearns, 1983). A large percentage of the research needs of the speech-language clinician involves development of new training or therapy protocols for purposes of correcting speech or language problems in children or brain-injured adults or similar patients. Single-subject experiments are used to demonstrate the effectiveness of a given therapy, as well as to determine which of several different therapies is most effective for correcting specific problems.

In the typical single-subject experiment, in contrast with the between-group design, each subject is used as his or her own "control" for purposes of demonstrating experimental control. If, for example, the experiment involves evaluating the effectiveness of a specific treatment (independent variable) for correcting a deviant pattern of speech production (dependent variable) in children, the clinician would, over a succession of training sessions, alternately administer and withdraw the treatment to determine if the individual child's speech production improved during sessions in which the treatment was being administered and stayed the same, or became worse, during sessions when the treatment was not presented. At the beginning of the experiment, the researcher would administer a series of baseline sessions, in which no treatment was presented, to determine the level of severity of the child's speech production problem. Subsequently, the researcher would begin alternating treatment and no-treatment sessions. If the child's speech production is observed to consistently improve when treatment is present, and to decrease when treatment is withdrawn, the researcher would conclude that experimental control had been demonstrated. The treatment appears to be effective in improving the child's speech productions. Figure 3–1 (*top panel*) shows graphed results for a typical experiment of this type. In performing an actual experiment, of course, the researcher would not terminate the study after testing one individual child. He or she would want to replicate the experimental control effect with several more children before reporting the results at a professional conference or in a peer journal.

The *ABAB withdrawal* design shown in the figure (in which A and B refer to the sequence of protocols used) is one of the more popular designs used in SLP research. Researchers who use single-subject designs have, however, developed a variety of other and, in some cases, more complex forms of single-subject designs for use in investigating specific research questions. For example, the *alternating treatments* design (see Figure 3–1, *bottom panel*) is used to determine whether one specific treatment is more effective or efficient than a second treatment in correcting a speech or language problem. In this design, instead of alternately administering and withdrawing a treatment, the researcher alternates each of the two treatments over sessions to see if one appears to be superior to the other in correcting the problem. For readers interested in further exploration of single-subject experimental designs, the textbooks by Hegde (1993) and McReynolds and Kearns (1983) are recommended.

In addition to the means by which experimental control is demonstrated, the single-subject and between-group approaches differ in a number of other important ways. The between-group design has its theoretical foundations firmly entrenched in traditional statistics and probability theory. Statistical tests are used to determine whether the experimental and control groups appear to be different. If statistically significant results are obtained, the researcher feels confident that the results from the samples tested in the experiment can be generalized back to the theoretical populations

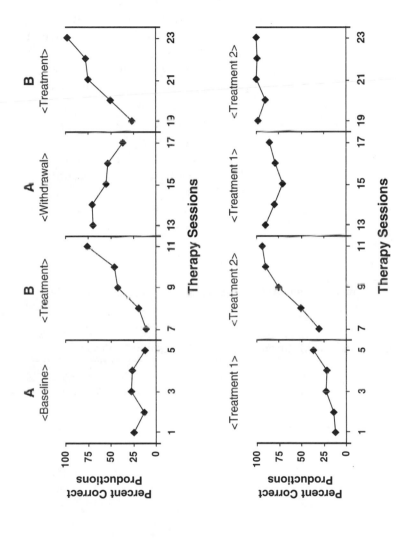

Figure 3–1. Graphed findings for a single-subject ABAB withdrawal experiment (*top panel*), and a single-subject alternating treatments experiment (*bottom panel*). See text for details of these experimental designs.

from which the samples were randomly drawn. The researcher then can predict that if additional subjects who are similar to the original subjects are tested, similar findings would be obtained. With the single-subject approach, the researcher typically does not use statistics to analyze the data and is not concerned with generalizing the results to any theoretical populations. Whereas with the between-group approach, very small differences between the experimental and the control groups may be *statistically significant* and therefore would constitute an important finding, with the single-subject approach, the researcher is more concerned with finding large *clinically significant*, rather than statistically significant. results. A single-subject researcher colleague recently quipped: "If you cannot see the differences in the graphic representation of the data at a distance of 30 yards with one eye closed, you probably do not have clinically important results."

Table 3–1 presents a brief summary of the strengths and weaknesses of each of the seven different research designs described in this chapter.

Table 3–1. Summary of strengths and weaknesses of basic research designs most commonly used in healthcare research projects

Type of Research Design	Major Strength(s)	Major Weakness(es)
Normative or case study	Good description of basic phenomena in field of study.	Indirect or direct evidence of cause-and-effect relationships is lacking.
Standard group comparison	Good description of specific differences between persons who do and do not exhibit specific condition (disease, effect).	Results constitute only possibly suggestive or weak indirect evidence of what the causal variables may be in cause-and-effect relationship.
Ex post facto study	Provides only indirect or correlative evidence of cause-effect relationships.	Strength of indirect causal evidence is dependent on how carefully study is performed, how many subjects are investigated, and whether test results can be replicated by other investigators.

Table 3–1. *continued*

Type of Research Design	Major Strength(s)	Major Weakness(es)
Retrospective outcomes study	Provides only indirect evidence of cause and effect. Design very similar to ex post facto except that studies deal more with clinical issues (e.g., treatment efficacy).	Strength of indirect evidence obtained is determined by similar variables as those in ex post facto research designs.
Prospective outcomes study	May provide direct evidence of cause and effect, because investigator has some control over causal variable (as in a drug trial study). "How good" depends on length of time between administration of causal and measurement of effect variables.	Because causal variables (drugs or treatments) typically are administered over long periods of time before effects are measured, this design often is susceptible to intrusion of extraneous variables.
Experimental between-group designs	These designs, if carefully controlled, can provide strong direct evidence of cause-and-effect relationships.	Strength of direct causal evidence is dependent on how well researcher controls for incidental or extraneous differences between experimental and control groups. Such differences may be the cause of the effect, rather than the variable manipulated in study.
Experimental single-subject designs	Because each research subject serves as his/her own control, strength of cause-and-effect relationship is dependent on how well study is controlled and how many times the effect is replicated with additional subjects.	Cause and effect may look strong for individual subjects, but confirmation of the effect or generalization to other categories of subjects (e.g., different ages, gender, educational backgrounds) is necessary.

CHAPTER

4

How to Survive the Tedious Data Collection Process

Whereas the research design dictates how the data must be collected, the research question dictates what specific types of data have to be collected. In healthcare research, all data must be observable and measurable, and the various types of data differ with respect to the mathematical scales of measurement they represent. To be valid as scientific evidence, the data must be the product of some kind of objective measurement. Although "subjective impressions" may be considered to have merit in clinical decision making, scientific evidence must be restricted to *objective measurements*. In almost all of the healthcare fields, including audiology and speech-language pathology, data typically represent either nominal, ordinal, or interval scales of measurement.

Most Common Scales of Measurement Used in the Healthcare Sciences

Nominal scale measurements yield data that fit into different categories or classifications. The numbers of patients who fall into different categories, such as those with and those without delayed language function, or those with and those without specific noise exposure histories, are data obtained using a nominal scale of measurement. Studies involving nominal data typically ask research questions such as the following: "Do more males than females exhibit presbycusis?" "Is the incidence of fluency disorders higher in males than in females?" Nominal data also are frequently referred to as *categorical data*.

Ordinal scale measurements yield data that also fit into categories, but unlike with nominal data, the different categories now reflect "more" or "less" with respect to some measurable variable. Examples are various types of rating scales (e.g., speech intelligibility scales, medical pain or discomfort scales). Different points (categories) on the scale indicate that something is greater or less than something else but do not indicate by how much they differ. Ordinal data also are called *ranked data*.

Finally, *interval scale* measurements are similar to ordinal data in indicating greater or less than, but now the different points on the scale indicate by how much one point is greater or less than other points. Examples are measures of length, weight, height, pure tone thresholds, vocal onset times, and so on.

Table 4–1 summarizes the unique characteristics of each of the three types of data.

Different types of statistical tests are used with each of the three types of data. Statistical tests that are used to analyze nominal or ordinal data are referred to as *nonparametric statistical tests*, whereas those tests that are used with interval data are referred to as *parametric tests*. Chapter 6 examines the differences between these two types of statistical tests and describes the individual tests most frequently used in healthcare research.

One common misconception that the relative newcomer to research may have is that "better"—more "sophisticated or scientific"—research requires that the project involve the collection of interval data, as opposed to nominal or ordinal data. Although it is true that more complex and sophisticated statistical test procedures have been developed for use with interval data than with the other two types, many important research questions require the collection of nominal or ordinal data. In the healthcare fields, the variables or phenomena of interest quite frequently represent so-called "lower" scales of mathematical measurement. The work of physicists and biochemists may focus more on the "higher" scales of measurement such as the interval scale, but this has to do more with the nature of the variables under investigation than with the sophistication of their

Table 4–1. Summary of three common scales of measurement used in data collection in healthcare research with human volunteers

Scale of Measurement	Characteristics of Data
Nominal	Frequency counts or total number of observations that fall into two or more independent classes or categories. The only mathematical relationship between the categories is "same" or "different." *Examples:* group memberships (e.g., male versus female), numbers on the jerseys of football players.
Ordinal	Distributions of raw data in which individual scores not only are "different" but also can be designated as "more" or "less" in relation to other scores. The numerical scores used in ordinal scales reflect relative position in the ordered series only and do not indicate "how much" of a difference exists between scores.
Interval	Data distributions in which the numerical values truly indicate by "how much" Individual scores differ from each other. The numbers associated with interval scales are quantitative and permit the use of arithmetic operations (addition, subtraction, multiplication, and division). Equal differences between points on any part of the scale are equal. *Examples:* age, height, weight, length, blood pressure.

fields. Many people would argue that studying the inner workings of atoms and molecules is a much simpler task than studying the "inner workings" of the normal or impaired language system.

It is important that the researcher, in conducting the research project, be aware of the type of data being collected. This knowledge not only will guide the selection of the appropriate statistical test procedures but will also prevent misinterpretation or overinterpretation of the "meaning" of the data. Although the simplicity of nominal data usually prevents gross misinterpretations of the meaning of the data relative to the phenomena under investigation, it is not uncommon for researchers to confuse the more subtle differences between ordinal and interval data. In my own observations, researchers occasionally may interpret ordinal data as though they were interval data. This is reflected not only in the use of inappropriate statistical procedures but in gross misinterpretations of the meaning of the results. For example, a patient who scores at level 4 on a speech intelligibility rating scale should never be reported to be "twice as intelligible" as another patient who scores at level 2. Although statisticians may argue among themselves as to how serious a particular instance of confusion between ordinal and interval scales of measurement may be with respect to the accuracy of statistical testing, the important point is to avoid such confusion in order to prevent possible problems related to data interpretation.

A not uncommon related problem occurs when the researcher designs a project that requires the collection of interval data and then uses inappropriate or inaccurate procedures to collect the data. This frequently results in a pool of raw data that do not conform to the mathematical requirements of interval scale measurements. If the data are then subjected to statistical analyses using tests designed exclusively for use with interval data, the results may not be interpretable or may even be misleading. It is absolutely critical, therefore, that once the researcher selects the appropriate research design and determines what kind of data needs to be collected, he or she must do everything possible to ensure that the data are collected in the most accurate fashion. *The quality of the research is only as good as the accuracy of the measurement procedures used in collecting the data.* A number of the more critical issues related to methods of data collection are considered next.

Calibration of Electronic/Computer Data Collection Devices

In recent years, audiologists and other healthcare professionals have begun to use increasingly sophisticated electronic instruments not only for making clinical measurements on patients but also in collecting research data. A similar technological revolution also is occurring within the speech-language profession, as exemplified by the recent introduction of computerized systems for evaluating voice disorders and other speech problems. At many university and medical center speech-language-hearing clinics, the same instruments are used for both clinical and research purposes. For legal and ethical reasons, it is required that all electronic equipment used for clinical treatment or measurement be subjected to rigorous calibration checks on a routine basis. This requirement also is critical for research purposes. If a researcher is planning to use a particular piece of clinical equipment for collecting research data, it is advisable that the equipment be checked and, if necessary, recalibrated at the *very* beginning of the study and again *immediately* on concluding the study. Many major pieces of clinical equipment are scheduled to be calibrated on a regular basis (perhaps at 6- or 12-month intervals) by the hospital's medical electronics department or the equipment manufacturer (or a designated service representative). If the equipment is not scheduled to have a regular calibration check for another 6 months, the researcher is advised not to assume that it is in calibration, and, if possible, to have it checked before beginning the study. If the research project continues for a long period of time (perhaps a year or more), the researcher may wish to have the equipment rechecked at specific stages in the study (perhaps after the completion of testing of different groups of patients) to ensure that no changes in calibration have occurred.

Sometimes the expense or time involved in performing electronic calibration checks on particular equipment items will preclude this being done as often as the researcher would like. With certain types of equipment, however, it may be possible to perform so-called *biological checks* on a more regular basis. If the equipment is the type that performs some type of calibrated measurement on a living person, an administrative or research assistant can be tested daily or perhaps once a week to determine whether the readings are staying stable. One person should be selected to be the designated "testee" for this purpose (at least until the person becomes "testy"). It usually is safe to assume that the testee's biological system will not vary much from day to day, so the equipment dial readings should show minimal variation. (In my experience with research involving measurement of research subjects' ability to detect certain types of sounds or discriminate small acoustic changes in particular sounds, my biological test subject frequently has been a healthy young administrative or research assistant. Periodically, I also use myself for these checks because the supposedly more sensitive and trained ear of the professional may allow the detection of subtle equipment problems that another test subject may not be able to perceive. Earlier in my career, I performed hearing studies with cats and sometimes even used an exceptionally cooperative and reliable feline assistant as the test subject for biological equipment checks. One such cat, who became a laboratory pet, was referred to as the "fuzzy voltmeter.")

Calibration of the Human Data Collector

It is absolutely critical that, in addition to having reliable and calibrated electronic measurement devices available, that the researcher or his or her research assistant be well trained and experienced in the operation of the equipment in order to obtain accurate data. The degree to which the human operator can inflict error into the measurements obtained with a particular piece of equipment will vary greatly. In some cases, the only thing the operator will need to do is push the buttons in the right order, and the equipment will do the rest. In other cases, the researcher or the assistant may need to make a judgment call regarding whether some event occurred or response was given. (In my own clinical experience testing the hearing thresholds of patients, even though a sophisticated and calibrated audiometer is used for this purpose, it is frequently necessary to make a subjective determination of whether the patient's response was "real" or not.) In many of the behavioral healthcare fields (e.g., psychiatry, psychology, speech-language pathology), the recording of subjects' responses is not as simple and straightforward as the hard-nosed scientist would like it to be. In speech pathology, for example, it may take the researcher many years of training and clinical practice to be able to accurately and reliably identify particular forms of pathological or abnormal speech production in patients. If the research project involves recording the incidence of certain abnormal forms of vocal productions in clinical research subjects, the investigator will either need to collect the data personally or have a research assistant available who also is skilled in making the same judgments.

If the raw data being collected in a particular study do involve elements of subjectivity or the possibility of measurement error on the part of the data collector, it is advisable to have more than one person independently collect the same data on the same research subjects. The researcher can recruit (or hire) one or more qualified assistants (e.g., graduate students or colleagues in the same field) and, if necessary, train them until their level of skill in accurately collecting data is reasonably close to that of the researcher. After the project is completed, the researcher can then calculate and report, as part of the final publication manuscript, a measure of *interobserver reliability*. These measures will indicate how closely the different data collectors agreed or disagreed in their recording of the raw data from the same subjects. Statistical correlations are a frequently used method of calculating such interobserver agreement. Many statistics textbooks (e.g., Hedge, 1993) describe this and other types of interobserver reliability measurements in great detail. The degree of interobserver reliability obtained in a particular study can provide research "consumers" with a basis on which to judge whether or not they can accept or believe the researcher's findings.

Use of Blinded Data Collection Procedures

If the data collection procedure does involve the possibility of measurement or subjective error, the person who collects or interprets the data may introduce a *bias* into the process. Unfortunately, an occasional less-than-honest investigator may deliberately misrecord or even fabricate bogus data in an attempt to obtain the most impressive (statistically significant) and publishable results. The newcomer to research must be made aware, however, that even the most honest and ethical of investigators can also, albeit unintentionally, introduce an element of inherent error to the collected data. For example, in an effort to be totally unbiased, the investigator may collect data or interpret findings in such a fashion that they are less significant than they should have been.

The solution to this problem is, whenever possible, to use a *double-blind* procedure in collecting the data. At the beginning of the study, a second investigator or a research assistant assigns a special code to each individual subject so that only that person knows which category or group (e.g., experimental or control) the subjects belong to. The investigator who then conducts the research study will have no knowledge—that is, will be "blind"—as to which subjects he or she is collecting data from. If the research project involves clinical interpretation of data previously collected from subjects (e.g., by x-ray examination, magnetic resonance imaging [MRI] study, or electroencephalogram [EEG]), another person must similarly code the raw data before they are interpreted by the investigator. Unfortunately, many research studies cannot be performed using double-blind procedures. The identity of experimental versus control subjects cannot always be concealed from the investigator who collects the data. In such cases, the investigator must be aware of the serious problems associated with unintentional biasing of the data and take all precautions possible to prevent this from happening.

One More Major Hurdle to Cross Before Data Collection

The atrocities committed by Nazi physicians and scientists in conducting human experimentation during World War II were the prime impetus for the post- war institution of rigorous laws and policies worldwide for the protection of human subjects. Before any research study involving humans can be performed, it must be thoroughly reviewed and approved by a special committee of experts to ensure that all volunteers will be protected from any unnecessary personal or physical risks as a result of participating in the study. Such special review committees are referred to as *institutional review boards (for protection of human subjects)*, or IRBs for short. By federal law, any "institution" (public or private school, university, medical center, or other agency) in which human research is conducted or promoted must have a duly appointed IRB panel to review any proposed research projects involving humans. All IRB panels use the same federal laws and policies to perform their function, including application forms and procedures, plus rules for the formal review and approval or rejection process.

The primary purpose of the IRB review process is to ensure that human subjects (1) will not be subjected to any unnecessary or excessive risks to their personal well-being (physical or psychological health) as a result of the study and (2) are thoroughly informed, in a written plus oral format, of everything that will be done to them during the course of the study including a detailed listing of any possible personal risks, however remote. A formal session is conducted with the potential research subject, during which the experimenter orally describes the details of the study procedures and risks, allows the subject to read a complete written description of everything presented, and then has the subject sign the consent form to indicate the subject is volunteering to participate. The experimenter and a designated third party witness also sign the form.

Subjects are always given a copy of the signed consent form for their personal records. Subjects also are carefully instructed that they have the right to withdraw from the research study at any time they wish, without any personal bias or negative repercussion from the experimenter.

Once the researcher completes the development of the proposed human research study, he or she will need to contact the local IRB office (at the sponsoring institute—school, university, or medical center or hospital) to obtain an IRB application package. Such packages contain formal application forms and detailed instructions for filling them out and submitting them to the IRB office. The office probably will require the applicant to submit as many as 10 or more copies, to ensure that all IRB members receive an individual copy. The chairperson of the IRB will then personally review the application and submit it to two IRB members who seem to have the most expertise in the subject area. These two people will be responsible for reviewing the application in great detail and presenting their findings to the entire IRB at the next meeting. The other members of the IRB also will be required to read the application in advance and be prepared to make comments or suggestions. Whether or not the application is approved, the applicant will receive a thorough formal written review of everything the IRB members thought of the application. The application may be *approved* pending a number of required changes in research procedures, wording of the consent form, or the like, or the application may be *tabled* pending major changes and resubmission by the applicant, or *rejected* as unacceptable per current IRB regulations and rules. Once the IRB application is approved, the researcher is free to begin recruiting and testing research subjects. If the project lasts for more than 1 year, the IRB will require an annual progress report and renewal application. If any procedural changes are required in the ongoing project that may directly or indirectly affect the research subject's risk factors, the investigator must immediately develop a formal written document that describes the details of all changes being proposed and submit it to the chairperson of the IRB. The chairperson may personally approve the changes or submit the new investigator's proposed protocol revision to the entire IRB for the members' review and consideration.

CHAPTER

5

Some Tips on How to Combine Research with a Busy Clinical Practice

Issues Related to Money, Time, and Ethics

The three most common obstacles cited by clinicians as impediments to conducting research in the clinical setting are *ethics, time,* and *money.* Many clinicians believe that withholding treatment from control group patients in order to measure the efficacy of some new treatment with experimental subjects constitutes a serious breach of professional ethics. Many clinicians also indicate that their busy clinic schedules do not allow them sufficient time to conduct research. Frequently, these same clinicians also bemoan the all-too-common fact that time taken away from clinical practice means reduced clinic income. All three of these problems are valid impediments to some forms of research—but not to *all* research.

This chapter first explores why very real concerns regarding ethics, time, and money need not necessarily be obstacles to all types of research and then proceeds to suggesting ways and means of performing research projects that are specifically designed to minimize the detrimental effects of such obstacles.

As indicated earlier, the goal of all scientific research is to isolate cause-and-effect relationships among the different phenomena associated with a particular field of endeavor. In the healthcare fields, this frequently translates into determining whether a particular treatment "causes" effective or improved outcomes with respect to some disease or health-related problem. If the disease is one that is life-threatening or detrimental to the short-term well-being of the individual patient, then using that person as a control subject and withholding treatment would make absolutely no sense, and would definitely violate all known codes of ethics. In many instances, however, it simply is not known whether a particular treatment is effective, or whether one treatment is more effective than another. Earlier animal model studies, or other types of nonhuman research, may have provided clues pointing to one or another answer, but until research with humans is performed, the researcher will not know the answer for sure. Thus, withholding treatment in situations in which it is not yet known whether or not the treatment works does not necessarily constitute a violation of medical ethics. Of course, researchers must not administer experimental treatments in willy-nilly fashion and are ethically obligated to take all appropriate safeguards to ensure that the experimental treatment, whether or not it is shown to be effective, does not produce other forms of adverse or detrimental effects. Therefore, withholding or withdrawing treatment in order to demonstrate treatment efficacy does not always constitute an unethical act. If we had solid and reliable evidence, based on previous controlled research, that a particular treatment is effective, or that one treatment is more effective than another, then we would not need to conduct research. Research is needed only when we wish to obtain *unknown* answers to important clinical questions. Constraints related to time and money will sometimes impede this type of research, but the question of ethics is rarely an issue. It would, on the other hand, be highly unethical to continue using and promoting (as well as billing patients) untested treatments that may later be found to be ineffective or even harmful.

Many clinicians believe that conducting research takes time away from normal clinical routines, with a resulting loss of clinic income. To some extent, this does happen, although as shown later in the chapter, means are available to minimize these problems. In some types of research projects, the clinician can take data gathered in the course of routine clinical activities and use this information as research data. It also is possible to set up controlled research studies in which patients are assigned as they "come through the door" to different groups, which then receive different treatment protocols. Some time must be expended by the clinician in setting up or arranging these types of studies, and in monitoring their progress to ensure that clinic staff are executing the steps of the study appropriately, but once the study is up and rolling, each patient will double as a research subject, and little or no additional time will be required to execute the project. Some clinicians may have the impression that collecting data for research purposes is more tedious and time-consuming than collecting data for clinical purposes. This is an erroneous impression, because the collection of data to track or confirm the progress of a clinical treatment protocol requires the same degree of thoroughness and accuracy as for the collection of data for research purposes. Other clinicians recognize that they may be able to survive the data collection process without going bankrupt, but they balk at the idea of preparing study results for publication, on the ground that they lack the necessary time or writing skills. These concerns are not unfounded, because manuscript writing can be tedious and time-consuming. In many cases, however, it is not all that different from the writing of clinic reports, which the clinician must do anyway. As indicated in an earlier chapter, the clinician may be able to obtain help with the writing task from experienced colleagues at local universities or medical centers. In all likelihood, however, once the clinician realizes that he or she has obtained valuable new research information that may bring the admiration and gratitude of professional peers, the "pain" of writing a manuscript will quickly turn into "ecstasy"—perhaps not unlike that experienced by the birthing mother!

Finally, some researchers may argue that, even if the time constraint issue can be brought under a reasonable degree of control, their pocketbooks will still suffer because it is unethical to charge patients who receive "experimental" treatments. This is again true. Patients should be billed only for treatments that are known to be effective. The research process itself, however, may provide the solution to this dilemma. The money lost while the clinician is evaluating the effectiveness or efficacy of specific treatment protocols may be more than recouped in the future when the clinician is able, as a result of the research, to implement faster and more effective treatment procedures. "Faster" could translate into the ability to see more patients each day, and "more effective" could justify higher fees for services rendered. Research is the means of weeding out the ineffective and less efficient treatment protocols and establishing the validity of those that are more effective and efficient. When this happens, everyone benefits, financially as well as healthwise.

The remainder of this chapter presents a number of examples of how the busy clinician may be able to modify his or her clinical practice to double as a source of valuable research information.

Adding Research Protocols to the Routine Clinical Testing of Patients

With this in-house type of research, every patient who comes into the clinic is considered to be a potential research subject. If the person fits a predetermined set of criteria required for subjects in a specific ongoing research project, the clinic staff will ask the patient to volunteer for additional special tests in addition to the routine clinical procedures scheduled for that patient. In this manner, research data are collected on one patient at a time over periods of several months or several years.

The practice of Dr. James Jerger and his colleagues, formerly at Baylor College of Medicine in Houston, Texas, is an excellent example of a healthcare group that used this format in a highly successful manner for many years. Dr. Jerger was the director of a very busy audiological practice at Baylor College of Medicine in which hundreds of patients with various complaints and disorders were seen every year. For many years, Jerger and his colleagues were at the forefront of research and development of new and innovative clinical test protocols for evaluating various forms of hearing and communication disorders. When patients were admitted to the audiological clinic, they received a battery of established clinical test procedures for which they (or their insurance companies) were billed. However, in addition to the routine clinic tests, many of the patients also were administered (with their informed consent) some special "research" tests (for which they were *not* billed). The data from the research tests were then stored, along with test results obtained from earlier patients, in a special file (a filing cabinet in the earlier years, and later in computer files). After data on sufficient numbers of patients had been accumulated, the test data were statistically analyzed and the findings written up for publication.

The unique feature of this one-patient-at-a-time approach to conducting research is that the details of the research design and test protocols are established in advance. Patients are not tested in willy-nilly fashion. If, for example, the research study calls for a standard group comparison design in which the clinical and standard groups must be matched on certain critical variables such as sex, age, cognitive factors, or audiological features (e.g., audiometric threshold levels), subjects are assigned to the different research protocols in such a manner that, over time, equal numbers of patients in each category will be tested. Thus, at the end of a year or two, this one-patient-at-a-time approach will evolve into large between-group research studies in which all of the appropriate control procedures will have been implemented at the same time that the data were being collected. This research approach requires not only patience (plus patients) but continuing attention to the details of the research protocol as it is being implemented.

Making Outcomes (Treatment Efficacy) Studies a Part of the Normal Clinic Agenda

Clinicians sometimes wish to investigate the relative effectiveness of a particular treatment or evaluation procedure they have been using in their practice. The raw data for such studies may be sitting in the patients' folders, having been collected as a byproduct of normal clinic activities during the past several years. These types of studies should produce minimal interference with routine clinic procedures. The clinician, or a nurse or an administrative assistant, can collect the data during those periods, however brief they may be, when clinic activities are least hectic. As described in an earlier chapter, certain control procedures should be used to maximize the effectiveness of this type of research for providing evidence related to cause-and-effect relationships. If, for example, the clinician wishes to investigate which of two alternative treatment protocols seems to work better, the study should compare groups of patients who differ with respect to which treatment they received but who are equivalent with respect to other critical variables (e.g., age, sex, other health factors).

As another example, both of two alternative treatment protocols may be known to be effective, as indicated by previous research, but the clinician may wish to determine which of the two may be more effective or better suited for specific types of patients. In the communication disorders field, for instance, speech-language pathology clinicians may wish to investigate which of two alternative treatments for phonological disorders is more effective with children; audiologists may wish to determine which of several alternative procedures for the fitting of hearing aids works better with elderly persons. Thus, the alternative treatment protocols are known to work, but which of them may be superior is unknown. In this situation, it would be perfectly ethical for the clinicians to conduct prospective outcomes studies at the same time that they are providing treatment to their patients. Using a one-patient-at-a-time strategy, individual patients could be entered into each of the alternative treatment protocols over a period of several months or even years. Of course, as with the retrospective outcomes approach, the clinician, or his or her staff, would need to carefully monitor the patient assignments to ensure that, at the end of the study period, the different treatment groups would again be matched with respect to other critical extraneous variables, such as age, sex, and so on.

CHAPTER

6

What Did I Find? Is It Real?

The word *statistics* has two common meanings: In *The American Heritage College Dictionary* (2000), *statistics* is defined as "facts or data of a numerical kind, assembled, classified, and tabulated so as to present significant information about a given subject." *Statistics* also is defined as "the *science* of assembling, classifying, tabulating, and *analyzing* such facts or data."

Healthcare researchers use statistics to achieve two major objectives: (1) to condense and summarize the raw data in order to more easily see any unique features, characteristics, or trends that may be present in the data and (2) to calculate the probability that these observed features or trends represent a purely "chance" happening or event. In achieving the first objective, the researcher (or the statistics consultant) calculates and reports a number of *descriptive statistics*, which provide summaries of the data in the form of various measures of central tendency and variability. To achieve the second objective, the statistician performs one or more specialized *inferential statistical tests*.

This chapter describes, in "nonmathematical" language, what the specific purposes of statistical testing are, and what statistics can and cannot do with respect to validating the results of a given research study. Also explained are the differences between descriptive and inferential statistics, and how the specific scale of measurement represented by the data (whether nominal, ordinal, or interval) dictates which of two basic forms of statistical tests, known as non-parametric or parametric tests, will be used in different analyses. Finally, a number of the more common types of statistical tests that are used in healthcare research are reviewed, also in nonmathematical language. This information is provided not to turn the reader into a statistician but to introduce the basic concepts and ideas behind statistics so that the researcher will be better able to communicate with statistics consultants, as well as to make sense of the statistical jargon used in published research articles.

What Can Descriptive Statistics Do for the Healthcare Researcher?

The function of descriptive statistics is, just as its name implies, to "describe" the data. After completing the data-gathering phase of the research project, the researcher is likely to have acquired a mountain of raw data in the form of page after page of numbers. The first step in the data analysis process is to try to get a broad idea of what the data may mean. The researcher must "assemble, classify, and tabulate" the data in order to identify any overall trends. This can be accomplished using one of two methods. The first method is to calculate some special *summary statistics*, which provide measures of both the *central tendencies* and the amount of *variance* in the data. In writing the publication manuscript, the researcher may include special tables containing all of the relevant descriptive statistics. If the researcher feels that the tables are not completely adequate for conveying the findings of the study to the reader, then he or she may proceed to the second method, *graphing* the data.

With the second method, the researcher develops and draws special graphs or charts that provide a visual display of the descriptive statistics. Numerous graphics software packages are available that will generate the graphs automatically when data are inputted directly to the computer by the researcher. Also available are a number of excellent combined statistics and graphics computer programs that will first perform inferential statistical tests on the raw data and then graphically display the descriptive statistical data in various formats. The different formats available for graphing various types of data are far too numerous to be included here. Essentially, however, most of the different techniques are variations of the three basic forms of graphs: *bar graphs*, *line graphs*, and *pie charts*. Figure 6–1 shows examples of each of these basic types. The researcher or the statistical consultant is likely to have access to these types of computer software packages and will easily be able to develop appropriate graphic displays of the data.

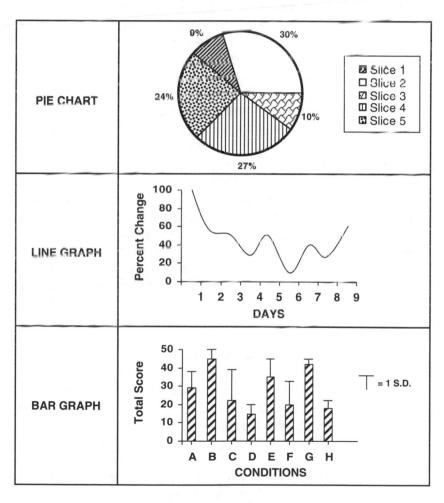

Figure 6–1. Examples of the three most common varieties of graphic displays used in healthcare research with human volunteers.

What Can Inferential Statistics Do for the Researcher?

Although descriptive statistics will show the researcher the basic trends in the data, it is the *inferential statistical test* that will indicate whether the trends *probably* are real or not. The key word here is *probably*. The basic premise or assumption underlying any inferential test is that the research findings observed in a given study are the result of pure chance. In essence, it is assumed that the same results would have been obtained had the researcher, rather than actually conducting the study, generated (contrived?) the data by simply flipping coins or tossing dice. A series of mathematical operations is then performed on the raw data to determine the likelihood that the results could have occurred by chance. All inferential statistics tests produce a *p value* (an index of probability, as described later on), which indicates the probability that the findings occurred purely by chance. A *p* value of .05, for example, tells the researcher that there is a 5% percent likelihood that the research findings are due to chance. Similarly, a *p* value of .27 indicates that there is a 27% probability that the results of the study could have occurred purely by chance. Later sections of this chapter elaborate on the meaning and interpretation of *p* value provided by inferential statistical tests.

As noted in an earlier chapter, the raw data collected in any given research study will conform to either nominal, ordinal, or interval scales of measurement. With both descriptive and inferential statistics, the specific scale of measurement dictates which of two basic forms of statistics, known as *nonparametric* and *parametric*, would be used in the data analyses. Nonparametric tests are used with nominal and ordinal scales of measurement, whereas parametric tests are used with interval data. Without getting into mathematical details, the basic difference between these two varieties of tests involves some assumptions that the statistician must make regarding the shape of the graphed curve for the *parent distribution* or *population* from which the *sample* observed in the research study was drawn. The parent distribution is a hypothetical concept that consists of *all* of the potential data that could have been collected (i.e., had the researcher elected to test every patient in the world!), and the sample is the data that were actually collected in the study (i.e., scores on the few patients that were tested). With parametric statistics, it is assumed that the graphed parent distribution is a bell-shaped curve (i.e., the data are normally distributed). With nonparametric statistics, the statistician does not have to make any assumptions regarding the shape of the so-called parent distribution curve. Thus, nonparametric statistics sometimes are labeled *distribution-free statistics*.

The parametric and nonparametric "equivalent" forms of the more commonly used descriptive and inferential statistical procedures used in healthcare research are described next. The goal of descriptive statistics is to provide numbers that will reflect the central tendency plus the degree of variability of the raw data. Different measures of central tendency will indicate the center or midpoint of the distribution of raw data values or, in other cases, indicate which data value is most typical. The different measures of variability provide numbers that reflect how "spread out" the raw data values are relative to these central points.

Measures of Central Tendency

Nominal data are data that fall into different categories or classifications. Accordingly, no mathematical relationship exists among the different categories—they are merely "different." Therefore, no measures of central tendency exist that can be used to describe this type of data. Some categories may contain more observations (data) than other categories, which will allow the use of inferential statistical tests (nonparametric) to determine whether the relative proportion of observations falling into each of the different categories differs from that expected by chance. With *ordinal* data as well, no measures of central tendency are available. With ordinal data, although it is possible to determine whether or not the categories differ from each other, it is not possible to determine by *how much* they differ. For a mathematically viable measure of central tendency, it is necessary to know the degree to which individual scores in the data pool differ from each other. This is possible only with interval data.

With *interval* data, the most frequently used measure of central tendency is the *mean*. The mean, which is a parametric statistic, is the arithmetic average of all of the raw scores. In certain instances, however, the mean may not provide the best representation of the central tendency of a distribution of interval data, as when the raw data distribution is skewed. A distribution of raw scores is said to be *positively skewed* when an unexpectedly small proportion of the raw scores have high values; when relatively more of the data have high values, the distribution is said to be *negatively skewed*. When the proportions of high and low values are similar, the data are described as being *normally distributed*. As indicated earlier, the "mathematically proper" use of parametric statistics assumes that the parent distribution is normally distributed. If the sample is skewed, the parent distribution probably also is skewed as well. Thus, in the case of skewed distributions, the best choice for a measure of central tendency may be either the *mode* or the *median*. These two statistics are the nonparametric equivalents of the mean and, as such, make no assumptions regarding the shape of the parent distribution. The mode is the data value that occurs with the greatest frequency in the distribution of raw scores or data values. Thus, the mode is the "most typical" data value. The median, on the other hand, is the score or value that represents the midpoint of the entire distribution of scores. One half of the scores will be above the median, and one half below the median value. Whereas the mode will always be a value that actually occurs in the pool of raw data values, the median may, on occasion, be a number that does not actually exist in the data pool. Most statistics textbooks expand on and clarify the specific procedures for calculating and interpreting these two nonparametric statistics. Figure 6–2 shows examples of normally distributed plus skewed distributions and illustrates how the mean and the median may give differing estimates of central tendency.

Measures of Variance

For the aforementioned reasons, no measures of variance are available for use with either nominal or ordinal data. With interval data, the three most common measures of variance are the *standard deviation*, the *range*, and the *interquartile range*. With both normally distributed and skewed data distributions, the *standard deviation* usually is the descriptive statistic of choice because it, along with the mean, is used in the more advanced inferential statistical tests. The standard deviation is a parametric statistic, whereas the range and the interquartile range are nonparametric statistics. If the researcher wishes to obtain a measure that more clearly reflects the actual dispersion in the data, then either the range or the interquartile

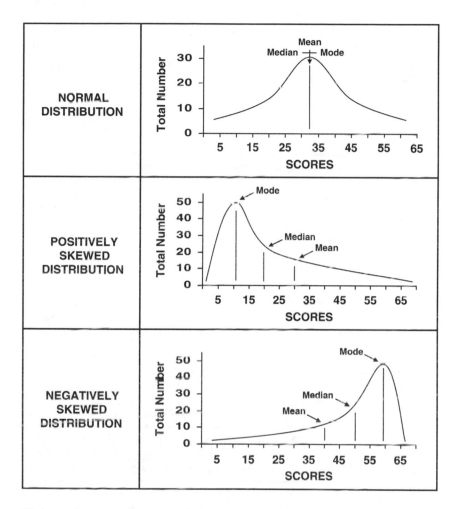

Figure 6–2. Graphic examples of normally distributed, positively skewed, and negatively skewed distributions of raw data, illustrating how the mean, median, and mode may give differing estimates of central tendency.

range may be a better choice. The range is simply the mathematical difference between the lowest and the highest scores. If, however, the data distribution includes one very extreme score, this statistic may mislead the researcher into thinking that the dispersion is greater than it actually is. In this case, use of the interquartile range may be preferable. This statistic determines the difference between the score at the 25th percentile from that of the score at the 75th percentile. This procedure avoids the problems associated with any extreme or deviant scores in the distribution. Table 6–1 summarizes the different measures of central tendency and variance.

Table 6–1. Measures of central tendency and variance for obtained research scores

MEASURES OF CENTRAL TENDENCY	
Descriptive Statistic	**Description and Usage**
Arithmetic mean (requires interval scale of measurement)	Mathematical average of all raw scores. Can be used when graphed distribution of raw scores approximates a normal bell-shaped curve.
Median (requires ordinal scale of measurement)	Is the score (real or calculated) that represents the midpoint of the distribution of raw scores. Is used when distribution of raw scores shows evidence of significant positive or negative skewing.
Mode (requires nominal scale of measurement)	Is the most frequently occurring score in the raw data distribution. Provides quick estimate of the most typical case in a distribution of scores.
MEASURES OF VARIANCE	
Descriptive Statistic	**Description and Usage**
Standard deviation (requires interval scale of measurement)	Is the square root of the sum of the squared deviations from the mean, divided by the total number of scores. Can be used when raw data distribution is normal or shows minimal skewing.
Range (requires interval scale of measurement)	Is the arithmetic difference between the largest and the smallest scores in the data distribution. If no deviant or extreme scores are present, gives quick estimate of total dispersion.
Interquartile range (requires interval scale of measurement)	The arithmetic difference between the score at 75th percentile and the score at 25th percentile. Useful measure of dispersion when extreme or deviant scores are present in raw data distribution.

The healthcare researcher usually is interested in much more than simply describing the results of the study. The researcher also will wish to determine whether or not the findings reflect real rather than chance effects. In order to do this, the researcher must turn to the use of statistics as a science, or as a specialized branch of mathematics. All of the different inferential statistical tests are the products of a specialized field of mathematics that is based on *probability theory*. The mathematical details of this theory are far beyond the scope of this book but are covered in numerous excellent statistics textbooks (e.g., Hedge, 1993). Probability theory is built around the critical concepts of *random sampling, populations,* and *samples.* To illustrate these important concepts, an example of a simple experiment is presented that contrasts how the researcher and the mathematician would interpret the data collection procedures and subsequent data analysis:

Research question:

RESEARCHER: "Does Drug X produce improved memory function in children with epilepsy?"

MATHEMATICIAN: "Drug X produces no significant changes in the memory functions of children with epilepsy." (rephrased in the form of a *null hypothesis*)

Step 1: *Enrolling study subjects*

RESEARCHER: Selects a group of 30 children with epilepsy. Then uses a table of random numbers or some other procedure, such as flipping a coin, to divide the children into two groups of 15 children.

MATHEMATICIAN: Regards this method of selection as random drawing of a *sample* of 30 children from the *population*, defined as "all possible children in the world, of the same age, sex, type of seizure disorder, same level of memory function, and so on, from which the sample (theoretically) could have been selected." Using a random procedure to assign the children to experimental and control groups guarantees two equivalent samples of 15 children who are still representative of that same population.

Step 2: *Data collection*

RESEARCHER: Collects study data as follows: Both groups of children receive a pre-test to measure their levels of memory function. Then one group (the experimental group) has drug X administered for a period of several days (or weeks); the second group (the control group) receives no medication or is administered some form of *placebo* (a pill containing some inert substance, such as sugar, rather than the drug). Finally, both groups receive a post-test to measure changes in memory function.

MATHEMATICIAN: Maintains that the two groups are still representative of the same initial (theoretical) population. Continues to assume that the null hypothesis related to the drug effect is true until sufficient evidence is obtained indicating that it "probably" is not true. (Predicts that the drug will not significantly change the post-test memory scores of the experimental children.)

Step 3: *Data analysis*

RESEARCHER: Performs statistical analysis (e.g., a *t*-test) to determine the degree of change in the post-test memory scores of the two groups of children. Finds that the mean test score of the experimental group shows significantly ($p < .05$) greater improvement than did that of the control group.

MATHEMATICIAN: Reluctantly admits (from an inherently conservative perspective) that the evidence is sufficient to reject the null hypothesis, which predicts no differences between the two groups with respect to the effects of drug X on memory scores. In essence, this revises former assumption about the study sample: Now, the group that received the drug actually represents a sample that was drawn from a different theoretical population from the sample that received no drug treatment.

On the basis of this conclusion, the mathematician would now predict that *any* epileptic child in the world who receives drug X probably will exhibit a similar change in memory function (i.e., the drug effect observed in the experiment probably is real and not due to chance). Thus, from the mathematician's viewpoint, the purpose of an inferential statistical test is to calculate the *probability* that the experimental and control groups were both randomly drawn from the same population. The p value calculated with the test provides this estimate. A p value of .05 indicates a 5% probability that the two groups are representative of the same population. This p value also indicates a 95% probability that the two groups are representative of two different populations, and that the differences observed between the two groups are real and not due to chance. (The mathematician, true to a well-deserved reputation as hard-liner, probably would try to get in the last word and point out the very real 5% chance that the mathematician is right and the experimenter is wrong. The mathematician might ask for a "recount" in the form of an independent replication of the original study by a second group of investigators.)

The most common inferential statistical tests used with each major type of research question are described next.

Two-Group Comparisons

The *two-group comparison* is by far the most common type of study performed in healthcare research. Many of the research designs discussed in Chapter 3 involve comparisons of two different groups of subjects. If, for example, the design is a standard group comparison, the researcher would compare a clinical group to a nonclinical standard group. If, on the other hand, the research design is experimental in nature, the study would involve the comparison of an experimental group with a control group. In this case, the experimental group may receive some treatment, while the control group receives no treatment. The researcher compares the two groups on some dependent measure to see if the treatment made a difference or not. For example, the researcher may be interested in seeing if drug X speeds up the mending of broken bones in children. A group of children with broken legs (or arms) would be selected who are then administered the drug. The researcher then determines the mean (average) number of days required for the limbs to heal. A second group of children also would be selected who are of similar mean age, health status, and so on, and who are similar to the first group in having equivalent broken limbs. This control group does not receive the drug. The researcher then determines the mean number of days required for this second group of children to heal. The researcher then uses a statistical test to determine if the mean number of days required for the limbs to heal differs between the experimental and control groups.

With two-group comparisons, the specific type of inferential statistical test used will depend on whether the scale of measurement represented by the data is nominal, ordinal, or interval. Some tests commonly used with each type of data are briefly described next.

With *nominal data*, the researcher typically is interested in determining whether the proportion of cases falling into two categories (i.e., groups) are different. For example, at Podunk University, do significantly more females than males enroll in Biology 101 courses? The inferential statistical test to answer this question is the *chi-square test*, or X^2 test (Siegel, 1956). By chance, equal numbers of males and females would be expected to enroll in the courses (for the purposes of this discussion, the small difference in male/female birth rates in the population would need to be ignored, of course). The X^2 test would test whether the actual observed difference in the male versus female enrollment totals differed from that expected by chance (i.e., differed from the predicted null hypothesis of "no difference").

With *ordinal data*, the most frequently used inferential test for comparing two groups is the *Mann-Whitney U test* (Siegel, 1956). With this test, the statistician first rank-orders all of the data from both groups from the lowest to the highest. The test then determines whether the rank scores of one of the two groups is significantly more clustered toward the upper end of the distribution than is the case with the other group. By chance, it would be expected that the individual ranks of the two groups would overlap each other with little or no difference in the "averaged" ranks.

With *interval data*, the *t-test for independent samples* (Runyan & Haber, 1976) is the most frequently used inferential procedure for comparing two groups. The *t*-test, being a parametric test, assumes that the parent distributions or populations from which the samples were drawn are normally distributed. The researcher needs to inspect the distribution of the raw data from the two groups to determine whether they appear to be skewed (see Figure 6–1 for examples of skewed and normally distributed sample data). The *t*-test can still be used if the data distributions are only mildly skewed. The researcher's statistical consultant will need to make the decision of whether the degree of skewing in the data is serious enough to contraindicate using the *t*-test. The Mann-Whitney U test is considered by most statisticians to be a viable alternative to the *t*-test as a procedure for comparing two groups whenever the raw data distributions indicate the presence of excessive degrees of skewing.

The statistics consultant also will be familiar with several special mathematical techniques that can be used to correct for the skewing in interval data. These procedures involve submitting the raw data to special mathematical manipulations or transformations and then using traditional parametric statistical procedures to analyze the mathematically altered data. The statistics consultant will need to determine whether such data transformations are appropriate with the researcher's data, or whether the use of nonparametric statistical tests would be the preferred means of analyzing the data.

Before-and-After Comparisons

In certain instances, the researcher, instead of wishing to compare two different groups on some dependent measure, may wish to compare the same group of subjects on the same dependent measure, perhaps before and after the administration of some particular treatment. The study described earlier in which the researcher wished to investigate whether memory scores of epileptic children changed after administration of drug X is an example of this type of comparison. If the data are of the interval type (and not badly skewed), the researcher, instead of using the *t*-test for independent samples, could use a different form of *t*-test referred to as the *t-test for correlated samples* (Runyan & Haber, 1976).

If the data are of the ordinal type, or if the interval data are considered to be too skewed to warrant using the *t*-test for correlated samples, the researcher may opt to use the nonparametric *sign test* (Siegel, 1956) for making before-and-after comparisons. The sign test determines the mathematical sign of the differences on the individual pre- and post-test scores—that is, whether the post-test score is greater (+) or less (–) than the pre-test score—and evaluates whether there is a significant difference in the proportion of the two signs.

Multigroup Comparisons

The two varieties of the multigroup comparison design are (1) *one-way multigroup comparisons* and (2) *factorial multigroup comparisons* (see Winer, 1991, for a thorough description of various parametric and nonparametric analysis of variance [ANOVA] designs). One-way comparisons are a simple extension of the basic two-group designs. In the example cited earlier, in which the researcher wished to evaluate whether a particular drug facilitated the mending of broken bones, if the researcher further wished to compare a second or even a third drug with the first drug, two or three experimental groups would be established, and the results for these groups would be compared with those for the control group that received no drug treatment. To analyze these data, the researcher would first use a *one-way ANOVA*. If this test yielded statistically significant results (i.e., in technical jargon, a significant *main effect* or *F-ratio*), the researcher would then need to perform further special statistical tests to determine which of the drug groups differed from the control group as well as whether one drug may have been superior to the others in facilitating mending. If the result of the one-way ANOVA test is not statistically significant (i.e., the *p* value is greater than .05), the researcher does not need to perform any additional statistical tests. A nonsignificant *main effect* indicates that there is no evidence that any group differed from any other group. A significant one-way ANOVA result (i.e., $p < .05$) tells the researcher that some of the groups differed statistically from the others. It will be necessary to statistically compare the results from individual pairs of subject groups to determine which groups differed from each other. These latter tests are frequently referred to in the research literature as *post hoc comparisons* or *paired comparisons*. The *t*-test for independent samples is only one type of post hoc test frequently used. Other frequently used tests include the *Sheffe test* (Schiavetti & Metz, 2002) and the *Tukey HSD (honestly significant difference) test* (Schiavetti & Metz, 2002).

The Problem with Using Multiple t-Tests

Use of the *t*-test for multiple-group comparisons is associated with the potential for very real problems with interpretation of data. Readers of scientific journals may encounter articles in which the authors, instead of performing ANOVA tests, opted to use a series of *t*-tests to examine the differences between each of several pairs of subject groups. As mentioned earlier, the *t*-test also is sometimes used for purposes of performing a series of post hoc comparisons. The use of multiple *t*-tests for either of these purposes may create special problems. Whenever a researcher uses several *t*-tests in a given study, he or she faces the very real possibility of obtaining results that appear to be statistically significant but actually are due to pure chance. If, for example, the researcher chooses a p value of .05 for the significance level and performs 20 t-tests in a study, 1 of the 20 t-tests is likely to yield a *false* or *spurious* indication of a significant result! A .05 significance level indicates that each time a t-test is performed, there is a 1 in 20 probability that the results will appear to be real when they actually are due to chance. To avoid this problem, it is recommended that if the researcher plans to perform more than five separate group comparisons in a study, the one-way ANOVA should be used first; then, if significant main effects are found, the researcher can use the Tukey, Sheffe, or another of the specialized post hoc tests that have built-in mathematical safeguards that reduce the likelihood of obtaining spuriously significant results.

The second form of multigroup comparison, the *factorial design*, is more complex and difficult to execute, but has the potential to yield more valuable research information. To illustrate this type of design, the earlier "broken limb" example is again useful. Now the researcher wishes to compare two drugs with respect to facilitating broken bone mending. The researcher also is interested in determining if the age of the patient is a factor in the effectiveness of these two drugs. So the researcher decides to look at three age groups—children, middle-aged (MA) adults, and elderly adults—with respect to how they respond to the two drugs. For this study, six groups of experimental subjects are required, as illustrated in Table 6–2.

In this design, half of the children would receive drug 1 and half drug 2. Likewise, half of the MA adults would receive drug 1 and half drug 2, and also likewise for the elderly adults. In the

Table 6–2. Example of factorial design for multigroup comparison: 2 × 3 factorial design

Patient Age	DRUG TREATMENT	
	Drug 1	**Drug 2**
Children	$n = 10$	$n = 10$
MA adults	$n = 10$	$n = 10$
Elderly adults	$n = 10$	$n = 10$

research literature, this design would be referred to as a *2 × 3 factorial design* (read as "2 by 3 factorial design"). The researcher would have two levels of the drug treatment variable (drug 1 versus drug 2) and three levels of the age variable (children versus MA adults versus elderly adults). Because two variables—age and drug treatment—are being investigated at the same time, the researcher would perform a *two-way ANOVA* for the statistical analysis. The ANOVA would provide two pieces of information, referred to as *main effects* and *interaction effects*. The statistical test would provide separate *F-ratios* for each of these two effects. Main effects indicate whether statistically significant differences between the levels of one variable are present, independent of which level of the other variable was present. For example, in the foregoing example, a significant main effect for drug treatment would tell the researcher that the effects of the two drugs probably are different—and that this difference does not depend on the age of the patients. Similarly, a significant main effect for patient age would indicate that the speed of broken bone mending differs significantly among the three age groups—and that this effect is independent of which drug was administered. Of course, in this latter case, because three age groups are involved, the researcher would need to perform post hoc comparisons to determine which groups differed from each other.

The possibility of finding significant *interaction effects* is a feature of factorial designs that makes this approach extremely valuable in healthcare research. A significant interaction effect tells the researcher that the effects of one variable (age or drug treatment) are dependent on which level of the other variable is present. In the foregoing example, a significant age-drug treatment interaction effect would indicate that which of the two drugs was superior to the other is dependent on the age of the patient. Drug 1 may be superior to drug 2 in facilitating bone mending in children, whereas drug 2 may be superior in elderly patients. With this information, the physician would know to use drug 1 only with children and drug 2 only with elderly adults.

Repeated Measures in Multigroup Comparisons

In the foregoing examples, the researcher used different groups of subjects with each of the different combinations of the drug and age variables. This type of design is referred to as a *completely randomized ANOVA* design (Winer, 1991). Thus, in the study of broken bone mending described earlier, the researcher needed to recruit a total of 60 research subjects. In some instances, however, the researcher may administer all levels of one variable to each of the subjects. This type of design is labeled a *repeated measures ANOVA design* (Winer, 1991). This was not possible in the preceding example because the researcher would have no way of comparing the effects of drug 1 and drug 2 within the same individual subject. If, however, the researcher had a "magic" x-ray machine that could accurately measure the speed of bone mending while the subject was taking a particular drug, a possible protocol would be to administer drug 1 for perhaps 2 weeks and obtain a measure of the speed of mending, and then administer drug 2 for the next 2 weeks and get a second speed-of-mending measurement. In this case, the drug variable would become a *repeated measures variable*, whereas the age variable would remain a between-group variable as before. The repeated measures ANOVA test would provide, like its completely randomized ANOVA counterpart, F-ratios for both main effects and interaction effects. If the researcher is performing a multigroup comparison that does involve repeated measures over one or more variables, it is critical that he or she select a repeated measures ANOVA test, rather than a randomized ANOVA test, because the mathematics and underlying assumptions of the two tests are different. Table 6–3 shows examples of "ANOVA summary tables," as might be depicted in published research articles, presenting the results of completely randomized ANOVA and repeated measures ANOVA tests.

One additional important form of *control* that researchers need to use when performing repeated measures, as opposed to randomized ANOVA designs, bears mentioning. With repeated measures designs, it is critical that the order of presentation of the different variables (e.g., drug 1 or drug 2) be counterbalanced from one research subject to the next. One half of the subjects should receive the first level of the variable first (i.e., drug 1); the other half of the subjects should receive the second level (drug 2) first. This procedure controls for any possible *carry-over effects* associated with going from one variable to the next.

The aforementioned 2 × 3 ANOVA designs involved only two variables. Such designs frequently are referred to in the research

Table 6–3. Typical summary tables for a completely randomized two-way ANOVA test and a two-way repeated measures ANOVA test*

SUMMARY TABLE: RANDOMIZED TWO-WAY ANOVA

Data Source	Sum of Squares	df	Mean Squares	F-Ratio	Prob.
Factor A	5602.81	1	5602.81	**24.35**	**<.0001**
Factor B	1963.10	1	1963.10	**8.53**	**.005**
A × B	580.33	1	580.33	**2.52**	**.18**
Within cell	12883	56	230.05		

SUMMARY TABLE: TWO-WAY REPEATED MEASURES ANOVA

Data Source	Sum of Squares	df	Mean Squares	F-Ratio	Prob.
Between groups	81.93	29			
Factor A	11.43	2	5.72	**2.19**	**.13**
Sub W. group**	70.5	27	2.61		
Factor B	29.40	1	29.40	**16.57**	**.0004**
A × B	.70	2	.35	**.20**	**.82**
B × sub W. group	47.90	27	1.77		
Total	159.93	59			

*Highlighted in **bold** type are the F-ratios and p value associated with the main effects of the two variables (factors A and B), as well as the interaction effects (A × B).
**Subjects within group.
Abbreviations: ANOVA, analysis of variance; df, degrees of freedom; Prob., probability (P values).

literature as *two-way designs*. It is possible for ANOVA designs to involve additional variables, in which case they would be designated *three-way, four-way, five-way*, and so on, ad nauseam. In addition to increased numbers of main effects, these latter analyses also provide results related to multiple and more complex forms of interaction effects. A three-way ANOVA would, in addition to three main effects, provide F-ratios for three two-way interaction effects (involving, respectively, the first and second variables, the first and third variables, and the second and third variables), as well as a three-way interaction effect (involving all three variables). A four-way or five-way ANOVA would produce even more complex results! These larger and more complex designs, in addition to requiring rapidly increasing numbers of research subjects, also frequently become unwieldy and difficult to interpret, as borne out by my own experience: For my PhD dissertation research study, I performed a six-way completely randomized ANOVA. This study involved testing 300 white rats in a very complex visual/somatosensory discrimination learning task. The ANOVA found a very puzzling but highly significant ($p < .001$) six-way interaction effect. After more than 25 years of head scratching, I have yet to unravel the meaning of this finding! Subsequent to this experience, I have consistently avoided research projects that require anything more complex than two-way ANOVAs. The newcomer to research would be well advised to do so as well. Simple studies are easier to perform and easier to interpret and can make contributions to the field that are as great as or even greater than those achieved with the more complex varieties.

Nonparametric Analysis of Variance Procedures

The one-way and factorial ANOVA tests require that the data conform to the interval scale of measurement. If the data are ordinal rather than interval, the researcher could select one of two nonparametric versions of ANOVA tests. The *Kruskal-Wallis one-way analysis of variance test* (Siegel, 1956) can be used to determine the probability that three or more independent samples were randomly drawn from the same population. If the research design conforms to a two-way factorial model and the data are of the ordinal type, the *Friedman two-way analysis of variance test* (Siegel, 1956) could be used. If significant main effects are obtained with either of these tests, special procedures are available to permit post hoc comparisons to determine which groups are different from each other (Siegel, 1988). Although other special types of nonparametric procedures have been developed for analyzing multigroup data, these are two of the more popular nonparametric ANOVA procedures in healthcare research today.

If the research data are nominal, rather than ordinal, two different versions of the X^2 test are available that can be used to perform the equivalent of one-way and factorial analyses. The X^2 *one-variable test* (Siegel, 1956, 1988) can be used with nominal data that fall into three or more independent categories of a single variable. For example, to determine whether significant differences in hair color exist among the students of a particular college, the researcher could select the categories of *brunette*, *blond*, and *red*, and then survey the student population and obtain a count of the number of students who fall into each category. The X^2 test could then be used to determine whether the relative proportion of students in each of the three categories differs from that expected by chance. If the researcher wished to further determine if any relationship existed between hair color and whether students were more likely to be in the top or bottom half of their class with respect to academic performance, a *two-variable* version of the X^2 test (Siegel, 1956, 1988) could be used. This test could determine whether there is evidence of any interaction between hair color and academic performance. If the researcher's data are nominal or ordinal, a statistician should be consulted as to whether a nonparametric ANOVA, X^2, or some other form of test would be most appropriate for use with the specific project.

As a research consultant, I frequently am asked the following question: "How large a difference do I need to see between my groups, or how many subjects do I need to test, in order to obtain statistically significant differences?" No simple answer to this question is possible. However, in general, the answer relates to three major factors: (1) How far apart are the means (or other measures of central tendency) of the different subject groups? (2) Within each group, how much variability is there in the raw data (e.g., are the standard deviations large or small?) (3) How many subjects were tested in each group? If the within-group variability is *large*, the researcher will need to see greater differences in the intergroup means (i.e., intergroup variability) in order for the effects to be significant. If the within-group variability is *small*, then smaller group mean differences will be needed to achieve statistical significance. Sample size also is an important player in this relationship. If the within-group variability remains constant, then as sample size increases, the researcher will find that smaller and smaller differences in the intergroup means are necessary to achieve statistical significance. Thus, in order to have the greatest chance of obtaining statistically significant results, the researcher should test large numbers of subjects, see very little variability from one subject to the next, and find large mean differences between the different subject groups. With hard work and effort, the researcher may be able to achieve the first requirement, and with "tight" experimental controls and careful data collection, he or she may even have some control over the second factor—but the third factor should be completely "controlled" by Mother Nature.

Fortunately, some statistical tools are available that can be used to prevent the new researcher from being totally dependent on the whims of Mother Nature when deciding how many subjects will need to be recruited for testing. A statistics consultant will know of and can assist in performing what are called *power analyses* and *estimation of effect sizes* (Keppel, 1991; Keren & Lewis, 1979; Steel, Torrie, & Dickie, 1997) with research studies. After the data are collected, the statistician will be able to analyze the test results to determine *effect sizes*—how big or robust the changes are in the dependent variable ("effect") with administration of the independent variable ("cause"). One version of these power tests (Cohen, 1977, 1988) calculates what is called an *omega squared value*, which will determine whether the observed effect sizes are large, medium, or small. If the researcher's initial study indicates small effect sizes, the statistician should be consulted regarding the possibility of repeating the study using larger numbers of research subjects. In addition to examining effect sizes after completion of a study, the statistics consultant also may be able to perform other special forms of power analyses on the research design (before beginning the study) that will allow the researcher to estimate how many research subjects, or how much data, will be needed to achieve effects of reasonable size, if they exist. If the researcher is performing research in an entirely new field that no one has investigated before, Mother Nature may still have the upper hand in determining the outcome of the study. The statistics expert may find that the usual power analysis "crystal ball gazing" trick just may not do the trick.

Correlational Research Questions

In the foregoing designs, the researcher administered some type of treatment (independent variable) and looked for effects with respect to changes in some type of patient measure (dependent variable). These types of designs are referred to as *experimental designs* because they measure the effects of some independent variable on some dependent variable. These designs are useful in finding *direct* evidence of cause-and-effect relationships—for example, drug 1 causes faster mending of broken bones in children. In many cases, however, the scientist's task is to attempt to obtain *indirect* evidence for the original cause or causes of some disease: The disease exists today, but the original cause is something that happened perhaps years ago. Thus, the researcher is faced with the problem of finding historical or anecdotal evidence regarding the original cause of some currently existing disease condition. The types of research designs used for these purposes are variously referred to (in the healthcare research literature) as *ex post facto, historical,* or *retrospective designs,* or sometimes as *medical chart studies.* The prior medical history of persons with and those without the disease or medical condition is examined to determine if *common factors* can be identified that distinguish between the two groups of patients. In some cases, the common factor is historical—for example, persons with skin melanomas are more likely to have a history of extensive sun exposure than are persons without melanomas. In other cases, the factor is some other characteristic or concurrent condition—skin melanomas occur more frequently in blue-eyed blond persons with fair complexions, for example. The statistical procedures used with these types of studies involve various types of *correlation analyses.*

A correlation test indicates the extent to which changes in one variable go along with, or parallel, changes in a second variable. The following statements are examples of such relationships between data: "As children get older, they tend to get taller." "As people get older, their bones tend to become more brittle." A correlation test provides a number or correlation coefficient, which can range from +1.0 to −1.0. A *perfect positive correlation* would be a value of +1.0. This would indicate that increases (or decreases) in one variable *always* parallels increases (or decreases) in the other variable. A *perfect negative correlation* indicates that increases in one variable are *always* associated with decreases in the other variable, or vice versa. A correlation value of 0.0 indicates that the two variables are totally unrelated, and that the magnitude or direction of change in one variable is completely unrelated to changes in the other variable. In the real world, correlations are rarely perfect. Typical correlation coefficients might be +.75 or −.75, or +.23 or −.23, and so on. Correlation coefficients of +.75 and −.75, for example, would reflect a stronger potential relationship between the two variables than would coefficients of +.23 and −.23.

In addition to giving a correlation coefficient, most computer statistics programs also will calculate a *p value*, which estimates the probability that the correlation value is a "chance effect" and does not reflect a real relationship between the two variables. The correlation values of +.75 and −.75 may be associated, for example, with a *p* value of .05, which would tell the researcher that "there is a 5% likelihood that the correlation value is a chance result." Likewise, the correlation values of +.23 and −.23 may be associated with a *P* value of .18, which would indicate that "there is an 18% likelihood that the correlation value is not real, and is due to chance." The *p* value obtained with all statistical tests—*t*-tests, ANOVAs, Sheffe, Tukey, and so on—are interpreted in exactly this same manner. The *p* value always indicates the probability that the results are due to chance. The smaller the *p* value, the smaller the probability is that the results are due to chance—given, of course, that the researcher used an appropriate research design and collected the data in a careful manner. By tradition, researchers and journal editors consider a statistical test result to be significant *only* if the *p* value is .05 or less. Some "hard-liner" researchers may insist that the result is not significant unless the *p* value is .01 or less.

Nonparametric and Parametric Correlation Tests

Depending on whether the data are of the ordinal or interval type, the researcher would use one of two basic forms of correlation tests. With ordinal data, the researcher would use the *Spearman rank-order* (Siegel, 1956) correlation test, and with interval data, the *Pearson product-moment* (Hegde, 1993) correlation test would be selected. Both tests provide correlation coefficients that can vary between +1.0 and −1.0. The Spearman value is designated as "rho" (e.g., rho = +.75); the Pearson coefficient is designated with a lowercase *r* (e.g., *r* = +.75). If the distributions of interval data show excessive degrees of skewing, the statistician may insist on using the Spearman rather than the Pearson procedure to calculate the correlation coefficient.

A Word of Caution In Interpreting Correlations

It should never be assumed that, because two variables are highly correlated, and the correlation is statistically significant (e.g., *p* value of .05 or .01), that the one variable "causes" the other variable. The two variables may be highly correlated *not* because they are casually related to each other but because of the presence of a third (perhaps unknown) variable that is the common cause of both variables!

A description of correlational designs would not be complete without a brief review of other more complex types of correlational designs. These other forms are referred to as *multivariate statistical methods*. Whereas the Pearson and Spearman correlation tests are concerned with examining relationships between single pairs of variables, these newer techniques have been developed to allow simultaneous examination of the relationship among *multiple* variables. These procedures have become very popular in educational and healthcare research, in which investigators frequently are concerned with identifying groups or combinations of factors (variables) that most accurately predict specific educational outcomes or the likelihood that a patient exhibits or will later develop some disease or medical condition. To illustrate the purpose and usefulness of multivariate tests, four of the more common forms of multivariate procedures are described next.

Multiple Regression Analysis

Multiple regression analysis is concerned with determining which subset of a larger group of potential predictor variables most accurately predicts the occurrence of a specific criterion variable. The technique involves computation of correlation coefficients between each individual predictor variable and the criterion variable, followed by determination of which combination or subset of the group of predictor variables best predicts the criterion variable. An educational researcher may, for example, measure a large number of predictor variables—scholastic aptitude test scores, IQ scores, personality inventory test scores, measures of extroversion-introversion, and so on—and then determine which combination of variables best predicts the student's school grade point average (criterion variable). The regression analysis may determine that the combination of intelligence quotient (IQ) and personality score provides the best prediction of (i.e., yields the highest correlation with) grade point, and that including measures of either scholastic aptitude or extroversion-introversion adds very little additional predictive power. On the basis of these results, future educators could limit total testing time per child by administering only the IQ and personality tests. In contrast with other forms of inferential statistical procedures, *multiple regression* or *multivariate* techniques are relatively new, partly because the complex data calculations and manipulations became practical only with the assistance of computer-age technology. Tried and true sources of information on this topic are the publications by Cureton and D'Agostino (1983), Monge and Cappela (1980), and Pedhazur (1999); statistics consultants may recommend others. Some multivariate techniques commonly used today in the healthcare sciences are summarized next.

Discriminant Analysis

Discriminant analysis is very similar to the technique of multiple regression except that the criterion variable, instead of being a continuous variable (interval scale), is nominal or categorical. This method searches for the combination of predictor variables that best predicts the subject's group membership. In the foregoing example, if the criterion variable had been "graduated from school" or "did not graduate," a discriminant analysis, rather than a multiple regression procedure, would be used. Discriminant analyses frequently are used in the healthcare fields to identify which combinations of predictor variables determine whether an individual patient will or will not later develop heart disease, cancer, or other medical problems.

Canonical Regression Analysis

Canonical regression analysis is similar to multiple regression in that it involves multiple predictor variables. Unlike multiple regression procedure, however, it also involves multiple criterion variables. The goal of canonical analysis is to determine which *set* of predictor variables best predicts which *set* of criterion variables.

Factor Analysis

Researchers sometimes measure a large number of variables in a single project (e.g., in a medical chart study). The factor analysis technique (Gorsuch, 1983) uses a complex series of correlation tests (which requires a computer) to identify any subsets ("clusters") of the larger group of variables that are highly correlated with each other; such subsets may represent different aspects or features of a more global variable or concept (i.e., a factor). In a sense, this procedure is designed to aid the investigator in characterizing the "forest" in which the "trees" are standing. Factor analysis has a long history of successful use in the psychological and education fields.

Table 6–4 presents an overall summary of the different inferential statistical tests described in this chapter, including which type

Table 6–4. Selecting the appropriate inferential statistical test

For Two-Group Comparisons		
Scale of Measurement	*Independent Samples*	*Correlated Samples*
Nominal or categorical data	Chi-square (X^2) test	No test available
Ordinal or rank data	Mann-Whitney U test	Sign test
Interval data	t-test for independent samples	t-test for correlated samples

For Multigroup Comparisons		
Scale of Measurement	*One-Way (Single Variable)*	*Factorial (Two or More Variables)*
Nominal or categorical data	X^2 test	X^2 test of independence
Ordinal or rank data	Kruskal-Wallis one-way ANOVA	Friedman two-way ANOVA
Interval data	One-way ANOVA	Randomized or repeated measures ANOVA

For Correlational Analyses*	
Scale of Measurement	*For Correlating Two Variables Only*
Nominal or categorical data	No test available (nominal data are "different" only—no mathematical relationship)
Ordinal or rank data	Spearman rank-order coefficient
Interval data	Pearson product-moment coefficient

*See text for multivariate tests.

of test is more appropriate for what type of data analysis. These tests are still widely used in the healthcare fields (and are the ones with which I am most familiar, having used them for many years in my own research). The field of statistics, like many scientific fields, is constantly evolving and changing. Over the years, authors of statistics textbooks have developed and presented other forms of tests that they believe are equally appropriate, or more appropriate, for particular types of data analyses. If the reader becomes involved in research, the statistics consultant may suggest using different tests from those listed here. However, it is important that the researcher select which test to use ahead of time and not be lured into the trap of "shopping around" for statistical tests that are more likely to produce significant results. This potential pitfall is described in Chapter 8 under "The Search for Statistically Significant Results."

CHAPTER

7

Writing Up and Publishing the Findings

The writing of the research article has a number of important and critical purposes, foremost of which is to sell a "product"—the researcher's study findings—to a group of very skeptical "customers"—the journal editor, the journal's manuscript reviewers, and, finally, the researcher's own professional peers. The researcher also will have to describe the study methodology in sufficient detail that it could be replicated by other researchers. All of this has to be done "on the head of a pin," because severe space limitations in today's healthcare journals usually force the editors to severely restrict the length of the researcher's article. Thus, good research article writing is diametrically opposed to good novel writing. The researcher as author must conform to a scientific or technical style of writing, which requires brevity, detail, and conciseness. Although various journals differ somewhat in their editorial requirements for publication manuscripts, all healthcare journals conform to a common set of requirements.

This chapter presents a typical format used for the research article and describes how each of these sections should be written. The basic sections of a typical research article—Title, Abstract, Introduction, Methods, Results, and Discussion—are described next.

The Title

All journals specify the maximum length of the title, in some cases as few as 50 characters, including spaces between words. The title must, however, convey to the reader both the subject area being investigated and the basic research question(s) that were asked. If possible, the title also should indicate the primary result or finding of the study. It is important that the title give as much information as possible regarding what the study is all about, for two reasons. First, when readers of journals are skimming the table of contents of the journal or the reference list at the end of a specific journal article, it is important that the title "catch the eye" to entice the reader to look at the article and possibly read it. Second, with today's computerized databases (e.g., Medline), specific *keywords* in the title are the primary means by which articles are indexed or classified. If inappropriate keywords are present, the article may not be indexed correctly and may be missed in subsequent literature searches.

The Abstract

Most journals will require a short Abstract at the beginning of the article. In some cases, the length may be limited to no more than 50 words; in other cases, the researcher (aka, the *writer* of the research article) may be allowed as many as 300 words or even more. The Instructions to Authors section of the individual healthcare journal will specify the maximum length. The purpose of the Abstract section is to allow the researcher to very briefly state the purpose and importance of the study, describe very briefly the methods used (including test procedures, types of patients, and so on), and state the major findings of the study. An important point is that for a majority of the journal readers, the Abstract will be all that they will read. Thus, in addition to being a brief and succinct summary or overview of the study, the Abstract also must be written as a kind of advertisement to attract or lure the reader into reading the entire article. Most computerized literature databases (e.g., Medline) include the Abstract in its entirety in the listing. Thus, the person conducting a computerized literature search will see only the researcher's Abstract and will use this item as the sole determinant of whether looking up and reading the entire article would be worthwhile.

Specific details of methods or results should not be included in the Abstract. The researcher (writer) needs to specify the types of patients that were tested, for example, but does not need to specify the numbers or any other unessential information, such as the proportion of males and females. Only the general methods used in testing the subjects need to be specified, not specific details, such as description of test equipment or numbers of test trials. The writer can state that "statistically significant" results were found but does not need to specify what statistical tests were used, or what p value were obtained. All of this information can be spelled out in the Methods section of the manuscript. A good analogy to keep in mind is that the Abstract describes the forest, not the trees!

The Introduction

The Introduction must begin by identifying the subject area and specific problem or question that was addressed by the research study. It should next briefly review the most relevant earlier research literature related to the area, with particular emphasis on describing how the earlier research may have obtained incorrect findings, used incorrect methodologies, drew inappropriate conclusions, or simply failed to address a particular problem or issue. This critical review is intended to convince the reader of the importance of the question(s) that the researcher chose to investigate. At the end of the Introduction section, the researcher will briefly outline what his or her study was designed to do that is different from what was done before, and how it will advance knowledge in the field.

The review of the relevant literature does not need to be extensive. Any classic original articles need to be cited, as well as the most recent publications. Journal editors usually select persons to review manuscripts who are considered to be experts in the topic area being addressed by the manuscript. The manuscript reviewers probably will therefore be very aware of how effectively or thoroughly the writer has critically reviewed the relevant literature. The researcher needs to take care to cite all of the relevant recent literature. If recently published articles are not cited, the reviewers may conclude that the writer has not done a thorough job of reviewing the relevant literature, or is not as knowledgeable in the area as he or she should be. Some journal editors may, in order to conserve space, specify that only a certain number of citations be listed. In such instances, the writer may wish to focus on citing only those recent publications that do a more thorough job of citing the earlier literature. This strategy provides a combination of "primary" and "secondary" citations that will give the reader a more complete listing of the relevant literature in the area.

It also is critical that in the Introduction, the writer provide operational definitions for any technical terms or concepts that may not have a clear meaning for the reader. Unfortunately, much of the *technical jargon* used in various fields of science can have multiple definitions. The writer must make it absolutely clear how the term or concept was defined in the study. Also, any abbreviations or acronyms—for example, "dB" for decibel—should be defined at first use of the term, either in the Introduction or elsewhere in the text. The fully spelled-out term is given, followed by the abbreviation or acronym in parentheses—for example: "decibel (dB)," "magnetic resonance imaging (MRI)." Thereafter, for the remainder of the manuscript, only the abbreviation or acronym (e.g., "dB" or "MRI") needs to be used. (In my own experience as a "consumer" of research, I have too often encountered published articles in which the author failed to provide certain critical definitions. The result was quite confusing as well as frustrating.)

The Method Section

At the beginning of the Methods section, the researcher will state, in detail, the specific research question or questions that the study addressed. Next, the researcher will briefly and accurately describe the details of the research design, the numbers and particular kinds of research subjects who were tested or on whom data were collected, and then describe the details of how the data were collected, including the types of electronic instrumentation that may have been used, how data measurements were obtained, and so on. This section should provide the reader with enough basic information regarding what the researcher did to allow replication of the study, if this is desired.

Many researchers find this section to be difficult to write. On the one hand, the journal editor may insist that the section be short, whereas the writer may feel overwhelmed by a mountain of methodological details. New investigators may very well be confused regarding what details need to be included in the manuscript and what can be safely left out and still provide enough information to allow the reader to replicate the study. If the article represents a first report of research in a specific area, the researcher will need to provide more detailed information. If the article is a follow-up or extension to similar research previously published by the same writer, not as much detail needs to be included. The researcher can provide a brief general description of the procedures and reference the methodology sections of the earlier articles for more specific details. In some cases, the researcher may have used identical or similar methodologies to those used and reported by other investigators. In such instances, again, a general description can be provided, with citations of these other published sources for more specific details. If the procedures used differed in any major way from that reported in the researcher's earlier studies, or in those of other investigators, it will be necessary to specify the exact nature of these differences.

Some general guidelines regarding what kinds of information need to be included in the Methods Section and what can be left out or described in a more cursory manner may be useful at this point: If any part of the methodology, such as a test or treatment procedures, items of electronic instrumentation, or specific patient or subject characteristics, was pivotal or critical in determining either the results of the study or the nature of the conclusions, this factor must be specified in detail (either in the article or by reference to earlier publications). If specific methods are not pivotal or critical, the writer may only briefly mention them, or may choose not to include any mention of them. Unfortunately, the determination of what is pivotal or critical and what is not falls into the realm of a "judgment call" and is one that not all researchers will be able to agree on. If the researcher believes that a specific methodology may possibly be critical, it would be better to go ahead and include it in the manuscript. The editor or manuscript reviewers may be able to assist the writer in determining the relevancy of a particular methodological item. Another strategy (one that I frequently use) is to send a preliminary draft of the manuscript to two or more experienced colleagues and request a critical review. The help of these colleagues is always acknowledged in the final published paper.

In general, specific methodological procedures or items of equipment need to be described in more detail if they are unusual or not commonly used in research or, for other reasons, may not be familiar to the readers of the article. If a rare or unusual treatment or surgical procedure is used, it must be described in more detail than would be necessary if it were a more common and widely known procedure. Likewise, a particular piece of equipment, if rare or unusual, should be described in more detail, including specification of type and model number. If the equipment item is more common (e.g., tape recorder, audiometer), only a brief generic description is needed. Certain other procedures usually need only brief cursory descriptions. For example, the fact that a randomization method was used to form experimental and control groups of subjects needs to be specified, but the reader does not need to know the details of how the randomization procedure was developed. Also, the reader should be told that critical equipment items were calibrated but does not need to be told specific details of the calibration procedures.

Almost every research project encounters technical and methodological problems or glitches somewhere in the long trek from conception to completion of data collection. Most of these problems are corrected long before they become "fatal flaws" and have no permanent effects on the quality or accuracy of the final research results. These problems typically are not described in the Method section of the article. Thus, the formal Method section actually gives the false impression that the study ran smoothly without any hitches. If problems did occur that the researcher feels may have compromised the study in any way, they should be described in the Method section and their potential effects discussed in the Results and Discussion sections.

The Results Section

The purpose of the Results section is to describe the details of the research findings using appropriate descriptive statistics and to show statistical evidence of how valid or reliable the researcher's findings appear to be. The researcher will provide summaries of the research findings, using tables depicting means and standard deviations (or equivalent nonparametric descriptive statistics), plus figures or graphs allowing the reader a quick "visual picture" of the findings. The researcher also will describe the types of inferential statistical tests that were performed on the data and list the outcomes of these tests.

The researcher must avoid any unnecessary duplication of information in the text and that shown in the tables, figures, or graphs. The text should explain the findings, while the tables and figures should show the results. The text could, for example, tell the reader that "the experimental group exhibited significantly better performances than did the control group," while the associated means and standard deviations of the two groups could be shown in a separate table. The text would tell the reader to look at the table for the summary statistics—for example: "These data are shown in Table 1." Every table, figure, or graph must have a short caption that very briefly summarizes what is being shown. The caption plus the associated figure or table should stand alone in conveying to the reader what is being presented. Many readers will first read the Abstract and then go straight to the tables and graphs in an attempt to find out what the study was all about.

The results of inferential statistical tests may, depending on which type of test was performed, be reported in a separate table, such as an analysis of variance (ANOVA) summary table, or enclosed in parentheses in the text—for example: "The experimental group exhibited significantly ($t = 4.54$; df = 6; $p = .004$) better performances than did the control group." The specific format in which results of inferential statistical tests are presented, as well as the format for tables and graphs, varies widely among different healthcare journals. After deciding which journal to submit the manuscript to, the researcher should select some articles from recent issues of that journal to use as a guide in formatting the manuscript.

The Discussion Section

In the Discussion section, the researcher relates the study findings back to the original research literature that was described in the Introduction. If the findings differed from those of earlier published studies, the researcher will need to discuss why this may have occurred. In this section, the researcher will draw conclusions as to what the study findings "mean" in relation to the field of research as a whole. The researcher also should discuss what he or she believes is the next major step that needs to be undertaken with respect to future research. Finally, because science is critically dependent on both accuracy and honesty, the researcher must point out and discuss any methodological problems or limitations that may have prevailed related to the research design, the method of data collection, or other factor, and indicate how the problem may adversely affect the generalizability or validity of the researcher's conclusions. The researcher should never cover up any flaws in the study! As borne out by my own experience, this type of soul-baring honesty typically is viewed favorably by journal editors and frequently improves the researcher's chances of getting the article accepted for publication. Nobody, and that includes the journal editor, expects the researcher to be immune to mistakes! Scientists do make mistakes—and sometimes the product of those "mistakes" is a major discovery.

Format Variations and Other Considerations

The foregoing format, involving six separate sections of the manuscript, is the one that most frequently is required by healthcare journals. Some variations on this format, however, may be encountered. For instance, some journals allow the Results and Discussion sections to be written as one combined section (Results and Discussion), rather than two separate sections. Many writers prefer this latter format because it sometimes is easier and more efficient to link these two topics together in the same section, as opposed to attempting to split them into separate and distinct sections. Finally, some journals require the manuscript to include a Summary, Summary and Conclusions, or Conclusions section as the final section. In some cases, this section is required in addition to the Abstract; in other cases, it is required instead of the Abstract. Like the Abstract, this Summary or Conclusions section is where many readers will go first to try to get an overview or summary of what the article is all about. Therefore, this section should be written to stand alone in giving sufficient information to convey the "big picture" to the reader of what was done and what was found. If the manuscript also includes an Abstract, the author will need only to summarize what was found and what it means in this final section.

Finally, although this should go without saying, it is important that the grammar, spelling, and general style of the article be as accurate and professional as possible. With today's word processors, spell checkers, and laser printers, this requirement is easily achieved. A researcher who recognizes that he or she lacks sufficient skills to produce a manuscript without some help should not hesitate (or feel embarrassed) to seek assistance from a colleague or another professional. The offer of coauthorship or a simple "thank you" in the Acknowledgments section of the manuscript usually will be sufficient reward for someone's help in this regard. Even if the researcher feels capable of writing the manuscript without outside help, it is advisable to have a knowledgeable colleague read the paper and provide feedback about the manuscript's clarity, accuracy, and thoroughness. (In my own experience as an author, I have found that having a friendly colleague read my manuscripts frequently results in the discovery of glitches, misspelled words, obtuse grammatical constructions, and so on, that had escaped my eye. I also have found that setting aside a "finished" manuscript for a while may allow a fresh look on my final read-through, with the same types of discoveries.)

Although a multitude of excellent publications are available to guide the new researcher in writing research reports in each of the different healthcare fields, an excellent general source is the book by Weiss-Lambrou (1989).

The Manuscript Review and Publication Process

Researchers need to be aware that healthcare journals differ widely with respect to how *prestigious* or respected they are among professionals in a given field. The more prestigious or respected the journal is, the more difficult it is to get articles accepted for publication. The journal *Science* and the *New England Journal of Medicine* are two journals that are very prestigious. The prestigious journals always have in place a very rigorous peer review process, with a high rejection rate for submitted manuscripts. Other, considerably less prestigious journals may not have a peer review process in place, or their review process may be considerably less rigorous. Some of these journals are referred to as "backstreet" journals by professionals in the field.

It is in the best interest of the new researcher to always attempt to get an article published in the prestigious journals and never submit articles to the backstreet journals. In developing a professional resume or curriculum vitae, it serves the researcher far better to list a smaller number of articles that were published in respected journals than to show a large number of articles published in backstreet journals. Unfortunately, as discussed in the next chapter, researchers may find themselves in a "numbers game" in which quantity may take priority over quality with respect to publications. Nevertheless, the extra work that is necessary to get an article published in one of the top journals will pay off in the long run.

When the researcher submits a manuscript to a respected healthcare journal, the editor will send copies of the manuscript to two and sometimes three or more outside editorial reviewers. These reviewers are professionals who are acknowledged as having special knowledge and experience in the topic area(s) addressed by the manuscript. These people will critically read the manuscript and advise the editor as to whether they believe the manuscript would be worthy of publication in the journal. They may determine that the manuscript is not worthy of publication, or they may decide that the topic areas addressed would make the paper better suited for publication in another journal. If they believe the manuscript is publishable, they may recommend acceptance with minimal or only minor editorial changes. In other instances, they may recommend acceptance contingent on major editorial changes or revisions.

The changes suggested by the reviewers can range from minor to major with respect to the amount of time and effort the researcher will need to devote to revising the manuscript. If the researcher is lucky, all that may be required is use of a word processor to correct a list of embarrassing misspellings, grammatical errors, and other minor editorial glitches. In other cases, the reviewers may challenge or disagree with more fundamental aspects of the manuscript. For example, the reviewers may disagree with how the researcher interpreted the study data and ask for an alternate interpretation. They also may believe that the researcher used the wrong statistical tests to analyze the data and ask that the the the data be reanalyzed. Finally, the reviewers may even request the researcher to collect some additional data to clarify certain theoretical questions or issues related to the interpretation of the findings.

If a reviewer's criticisms or suggestions for revision appear to be valid and will improve the quality of the final published product, the writer should proceed with making the requested changes. If, on the other hand, the researcher believes that a reviewer's' suggestions are not valid, or that they misunderstood or misinterpreted some part of the manuscript, then the researcher has the right to submit a polite written rebuttal to the editor, who then send this written response back to the original reviewer. The reviewer may then either concede that the criticism was in error or may dig in and insist that the suggested revisions are still necessary. In the latter event, the journal editor must then decide who is correct and pass judgment in favor of either the reviewer or the writer. The editor has the responsibility of making the final decision regarding publication and may need to do so without a full consensus of opinion from the reviewers.

CHAPTER

8

Pitfalls to Avoid in Research in Humans

This chapter takes a look at some common myths regarding the nature of science and the activities of scientists and exposes the reality behind them. In addition, a number of common pitfalls related to research are explored.

The road to scientific discovery is not as formal or predictable as the science textbooks (and Hollywood movies) would lead us to believe. That eighth grade science textbook listing the "five steps of the scientific method" is fostering a myth. The scientist's brilliant discovery is just as likely to be the result of an illogical, stumbling thought process as of logical and systematic problem solving. Scientists are supposed to be highly critical and original thinkers whose only motivation is the advancement of scientific truth. Most scientists, in reality, are biased and accept the majority opinion (the prevailing *zeitgeist*—described a little later on) of the scientific community. Those few scientists who do challenge the establishment may incur the wrath of their colleagues, and their work may go unpublished and unfunded. It has been said, somewhat cynically, that the only way science advances is when the older scientists, who are the guardians of the current scientific model, die off and the younger radicals gain a chance to become the guardians of a new prevailing school of thought. As explored later in the chapter, however, the flaws inherent in human nature can be the source of considerable error in the conduct of research and interpretation of findings. Awareness of such flaws and their effects is essential for the budding new researcher. Especially in this context, forewarned is forearmed.

Some years ago, Theodore X. Barber (1976) addressed this and related issues in "Pitfalls in Human Research." Although written by a psychologist primarily for psychologists, this monograph presents an excellent description of the various problems that scientists encounter when conducting research. For the reader involved in performing behavioral investigations with human subjects, this monograph is well worth reading.

Some of the more common pitfalls that are encountered by investigators in the healthcare professions are considered next.

Effects of the Prevailing Zeitgeist

Although the scientist is supposed to be a free thinker with an open mind to new and novel ideas, most scientists are, in reality, quite anchored to what they were taught in school. The scientist makes numerous assumptions regarding "how things are" that reflect the opinions and beliefs of professors and mentors, among other influences. In many cases, the scientist is not even aware of these assumptions—which therefore can act as blinders to limit the scientist's view.

In all fields of science, there appear to exist two distinct levels of assumptions that affect the work of the scientist. The first and most pervasive level involves the more global concept of "how the world is." This level incorporates the prevailing *zeitgeist* (a German word meaning "trend of thought in a given period") or what Kuhn (1962) has described as a *paradigm*. Kuhn used this term to refer to a conceptual framework and a body of assumptions, beliefs, and related research methods and techniques that are shared by a large group of scientists at a particular time. The paradigm, by providing the overall conceptual framework, serves to define what is considered to be "acceptable" problems to be investigated, as well as similarly acceptable methods for conducting research plus acceptable ways of interpreting the resulting data. Thus, although the paradigm can act to benefit the scientific field by fostering intensive and focused research by a large group of scientists, by setting limits on what is considered normal or acceptable research, it also can act to impede the advancement of the field.

The history of science is filled with numerous examples of how existing paradigms both benefited and impeded science at the same time. In astronomy, the concept originated by Ptolemy and his disciples that the earth was at the center of the universe and that the stars, sun, and moon all revolved around the earth defined the prevailing paradigm for many years. When Galileo challenged this paradigm by suggesting that the sun was the center of the then-known universe, the authorities were aghast, and he was accused of heresy. Galileo was, on threat of loss of life and limb by the church, forced to publicly recant his ideas. In today's world, his challenge probably would have been countered by less physical means involving the threat of loss of research grants and tenure by the peer review system.

Kuhn (1962) refers to the replacement of one paradigm by another paradigm as constituting a *paradigm shift*. In physics, the replacement of newtonian physics by Einstein's concept of relativity involved a paradigm shift. The field of psychology has seen, over the years, a number of paradigm shifts variously labeled as *behaviorist psychology*, *gestalt psychology*, *skinnerian psychology*, and others. Unlike the more pervasive paradigms in astronomy and physics, those in psychology were more visible to scientists working in the field. This was due to the fact that, at times, more than one paradigm existed and each had a large number of disciples who waged professional battles with each other. The proponents of the different paradigms even staked out and defended their own territories in the form of separate professional associations and "closed" specialty journals.

The medical and biological fields also have seen a number of paradigm shifts including, for example, the shift from the concept of inheritance of acquired traits proposed by Lamarck and his followers to that of Mendel's concept of the separate inheritance of unit characteristics. For hundreds of years, the brain sciences have seen what can only be described as a continuing series of paradigm "swings," rather than shifts, between the opposing concepts of strict localization versus nonlocalization with respect to structure-function relationships (Luria, 1966). The contrast between Gall and his concept of *phrenology* and that of Karl Lashley's *equipotentiality* concept best illustrates the pendulum-like nature of the evolution of this field. Gall measured and mapped various bumps on the skulls of humans and assigned different and unique functions to each of the bumps; Lashley, by contrast, argued that all parts of the cerebral cortex participate in each and every function.

Although the basic assumptions associated with the paradigms of any particular scientific field tend to be accepted and not questioned by most scientists, a second level of assumptions associated with the infrastructure of the paradigms tend to be questioned and frequently challenged by researchers. Paradigms can be thought of as defining the skeletal framework for the whole field. The job of the researcher is to investigate and identify the individual parts or components of the paradigm's infrastructure. In this regard, although scientists tend not to challenge the basic assumptions of the paradigm itself, they may argue among themselves regarding the assumptions related to the paradigm's infrastructure. For example, the psychologist accepts the basic tenets related to behaviorism but may challenge specific theories related to the use of behaviorism to explain how a particular species of animal learns a specific discrimination task. The psychologist may remain focused on determining how the basic concept of behaviorism can be expanded or modified to explain the animal's behavior but would never consider tossing behaviorism out the window and shifting to a new paradigm to explain the behavior. Paradigm shifts occur very slowly and typically involve a combination of the dying off of the guardians of the current paradigm and propagation of the new paradigm by indoctrination of their own students by its proponents. On occasion, a major scientific breakthrough, or a radical discovery, may trigger a more rapid shift. Einstein's theories of relativity and their subsequent laboratory confirmations launched a major paradigm shift, as did Louis Pasteur's discovery of the role of microorganisms in human disease, or Marie Curie's discovery of x-rays.

Thus, researchers are human beings, and despite what we would like to believe, even the best of scientists can be closed-minded in some respect. Armed with these realizations, the new investigator can recognize where his or her own biases come from and may even become more open-minded. The new investigator must be aware of the influences that the prevailing paradigm(s) in their respective field may have on how well a particular research project will be accepted by their professional peers. The new researcher must be aware that the journal editors and peer reviewers to whom manuscripts will be submitted for publication are likely to be supporters of the current paradigms. Likewise, applications for external research grant support will be reviewed by review panels whose members probably support the current paradigms. This fact does not mean that the new researcher must become a conformist with respect to research ideas. A researcher who develops an idea for a research project that is likely to be in conflict with the establishment should nonetheless go ahead with the project. The researcher must recognize, however, that it will be an uphill battle to get peers to accept the research. The researcher will need to spend extra time and effort in making sure that all facets of the project (the research questions, design, methods of data collection, and so on) are as accurate and scientifically sound as possible. The publication manuscript for such a project must reflect the researcher-author's awareness that the study contains radical ideas or concepts and must focus on presenting a complete and convincing rationale and argument in support of the project.

How Biased Are You?

The reader is asked to take a quiz to determine how "biased" a scientist you presently are, or how "strongly" you believe in the truth of the beliefs that are commonly accepted by you and your professional peers. Please write out answers to the following questions.

1. With respect to cause-and-effect relationships among the different natural phenomena related to your immediate professional field, what are some primary assumptions—concepts, ideas, or basic "facts"—that you believe are accurate and true?

2. Why do you believe these assumptions are true? (*Select one*: learned it in school; read it in a textbook or journal article; got struck by lightning; encountered a burning bush)

3. Other than being told by your professors or professional mentors that the assumptions are true, are you aware of any published research that supports their truth?

4. Do you know of any published research that refutes or challenges the truth of any of the assumptions?

5. How would you respond if a respected colleague walked up to you and challenged the truth of one of the assumptions?

(*Select one*: punch the obnoxious fool in the nose; decide that the colleague is stupid/has lost a significant number of marbles/ needs to take additional training; consider the possibility, however remote, that the colleague may be correct)

The closed-minded scientist does not question his or her basic assumptions, or, even worse, fails to even recognize them as assumptions. Most people accept, without any question, what they have learned or been taught. The open-minded scientist recognizes the assumption as being just that, and is willing to tolerate or consider the possibility, however remote, that the assumption may not be true. However, human nature being what it is, the open-minded scientist will still be biased to some degree (some people more so than others) and will choose to believe the assumption to be true until it is convincingly proved to be untrue.

Responding to Publish-or-Perish Pressures

If a substantial proportion of the researcher's professional duties involve research, and the researcher is on the faculty of a university or medical school, that person will be expected to publish. Academic promotions, tenure appointment, and salary level will all, to some extent, be dependent on quantity and quality of the researcher's annual publication output. Although quality and number should be equally important for professional advancement, it is an unfortunate fact of life (or of the times) that the number of publications may, at some institutions, take priority over quality. Of course, the *quality* of a researcher's publications is difficult to measure. Some commonly accepted guidelines include (1) the rejection rate of the publishing journal (the higher the rate, the more prestigious the journal), (2) whether the journal is *refereed* (i.e., uses multiple peer reviewers to judge acceptability for publication), and (3) how widely circulated the journal is among professionals in the field. Another frequently used guideline involves how often the researcher has had his or her articles cited by other researchers in the profession. A monthly periodical titled the *Science Citation Index* maintains a count of how often and in which journals the individual researcher's work has been cited. Most university and medical center libraries maintain collections of this index. Computerized versions of this index also are now available that allow tenure review committees to examine the number of citations of the tenure candidate.

An unfortunate consequence of this publish-or-perish pressure is to tempt many researchers into sacrificing quality for quantity in order to survive in their professional careers. Many researchers will opt to perform several "quick and dirty" projects and publish them in so-called backstreet journals (those with less rigorous publication requirements), rather than taking the extra care and effort to publish the results of a smaller number of more carefully performed studies in more prestigious journals. The publish-or-perish policy promoted at many medical centers and universities has been, in my opinion, the single greatest impediment to the advancement of science. A person who wants to do research to advance scientific knowledge should be encouraged to do so by universities and medical centers. Conversely, a particular faculty member who has no interest in research should be rewarded by the system for achieving excellence in other domains (e.g., innovative teaching, textbook writing, administrative or clinical duties). Forcing a person to do research is a very effective means of "polluting the scientific waters"!

The Search for Statistically Significant Results

Many investigators, and especially the newcomer to research, have the misconception that, in order to get their research published, their results must be *statistically significant.* Unfortunately, this notion has been inadvertently fostered and supported by the scientific establishment. Barber (1976) cites a number of surveys of the publication policies of several well-respected psychology research journals in which evidence was obtained that many editors and manuscript reviewers do in fact have a bias toward publishing only manuscripts that report significant findings.

This publication bias is problematic in the sense that it also tends to trigger a number of unfortunate responses in some researchers. Some researchers may opt to *table* or not publish their findings for a particular study if the results fail to reach acceptable levels of statistical significance (typically, p value of .05 or less). They feel that the manuscript probably would be rejected anyway, so why bother to write up the results? Researchers may have the misconception that the finding of nonsignificant results somehow indicates that something is wrong with the study. They may believe that the wrong research design was used, that the wrong data were collected or not collected accurately, or even that the research topic itself or the research questions were somehow inadequate or inappropriate.

It's important to recognize that finding nonsignificant results in a research study does not necessarily invalidate the importance of the research. Of course, a researcher who selects an inappropriate design and uses sloppy data collection procedures is more likely to obtain nonsignificant effects with any given statistical test. If the researcher does use the appropriate design and does collect the data carefully and accurately, however, then even statistically nonsignificant results may provide important new information. If a researcher is investigating phenomena in an *unknown* area (which should be the case if the study constitutes true research) and asks important questions, then the answers to those questions should provide valuable new information, regardless of what the answers may be. If a clinical investigator performs a study to determine whether or not a new type of drug produces a particular effect in patients with a particular disease, then "yes" and "no" answers should be equally important. The finding of statistically nonsignificant differences between the experimental and control groups (i.e., a "no" answer) may not be the clinician's preferred answer, but it would be, for the researcher, a valid and important answer that should be published.

As noted in an earlier chapter, in setting up and conducting research, the researcher should determine in advance what design will be used and should specify which particular statistical tests will be used to analyze the data. Some researchers, if they fail to obtain significant results with their preselected statistical tests, will "shop around" in an attempt to find some alternate statistical test that will yield significant results. For example, if a t-test fails to yield significant results, the researcher may run a Mann-Whitney U test (the nonparametric equivalent of the t-test); then, if this test produces significant results, the researcher would then proceed with writing the publication manuscript and describing this test as the one originally selected to be used in the study. Whenever a researcher shops around to find statistically significant results, he or she encounters the same problem described in Chapter 6 related to the use of multiple t-tests. Whenever more than one statistical test is performed there is an increased likelihood that the researcher will obtain spuriously significant results—that is, results that appear to be significant but actually are due to chance. The more statistical tests the researcher performs, the greater the likelihood of this happening. Thus, a researcher who shops around long enough will be almost certain to find so-called significant results.

In their quest for statistically significant results, researchers also may fall into some other traps. For example, if the original calculation of the statistical test yields nonsignificant results, the researcher is likely to look for mathematical errors (or recheck the data entries in the computer). If the results are significant, the researcher may not recheck the data or the math. Also, if the researcher collects a large amount of data and finds that the originally selected statistical tests fail to yield significant results, he or she may then look to see if any pieces or parts of the data pool may provide answers to other research questions that are perhaps different from the originally intended questions. Thus, the researcher will shop around in the larger pool of raw data in an attempt to find something—anything!—that *will* be significant. The researcher then will proceed to writing a manuscript describing this "postmortem" study as though it were the originally conceived research project. The problem that this tactic creates is again similar to that described with the use of multiple *t*-tests. If the researcher has a sufficiently large amount of raw data, then he or she will be almost certain to find that some part of that data pool will yield significant answers to one or more research questions. The researcher who has collected large amounts of data should always first perform a more global statistical analysis of the data (e.g., ANOVA or multivariate analysis procedures). If this type of test yields significant effects, it is then appropriate to perform post hoc statistical procedures to determine if certain parts of the total data pool are different from other parts. The researcher must never collect a large amount of data and then proceed directly to "dissecting" or "carving up" the data in a search for statistically significant differences among individual parts. In this regard, an important point worthy of emphasis is that it is better to avoid complex studies requiring the collection of massive amounts of data. Such projects may be too complex to perform or to interpret effectively. The smaller, more manageable research study is easier to perform and interpret and frequently yields results that are as important as or, in many cases, more important than their more complex counterparts.

The Very Fragile Nature of the Research Enterprise

Throughout this book, the essentially very fragile nature of research has been emphasized. The primary goal of any scientific investigation is to obtain a *totally* accurate answer to the question(s) posed in the study. Some research questions cannot be pursued simply because, at present, we lack the technology (such as electronic instrumentation, for example) to obtain the answers. As technology advances, so does the scientist's ability to ask increasingly sophisticated and complicated questions. In recent years, for example, so-called space age technology has allowed the development of faster and more powerful computers, which has, in turn, allowed mind-staggering advances in such fields as neuroimaging. (So why do we not have a cure for the common cold?)

Although the scientist may have the technology needed to obtain answers to the research questions, numerous sources of known and unknown pitfalls that can invalidate the results of any given research project still exist. Previous chapters have described many such pitfalls. The research designs that are used to investigate different questions all have inherent limitations and weaknesses. The experimental design may be the strongest design with respect to obtaining more direct evidence for cause-and-effect relationships, but as we have seen, this design also is quite fragile. In order for this design to work, the researcher must carefully implement a large number of control procedures. Without proper selection and use of such procedures (e.g., matching experimental and control subjects on incidental or extraneous variables), the results of the study may be worthless. The nonexperimental designs are even more fragile in this respect. In many cases, with these designs the researcher is not able to implement the control procedures that are needed and must trust that extraneous variables are not present.

Also, most newcomers to research and, unfortunately, many veteran researchers place far too much faith in the ability of statistics to "validate" the results of the research project. At best, statistics can serve as nothing more than a "neutral referee" to assist the researcher in obtaining a very rough estimate of the likelihood that their findings are the result of chance effects. The statistical test will perform the same mathematical calculations and give the same p value regardless of whether or not the researcher used the proper research design, implemented the necessary control procedures or conditions, or collected the data in a careful fashion (again, the relevance of "garbage in, garbage out!" is evident). The researcher must keep this critical limitation of the use of statistics clearly in mind. If the researcher does the proper footwork in designing and conducting the research, then statistics will assist in validating their results; without this footwork, then statistics may very well assist the researcher in "polluting the scientific waters"!

Because of the very fragile nature of research with respect to finding the truth, how can the individual researcher know whether his or her own or someone else's research is accurate or not? No simple answer to this question has been identified. The following suggestions, however, are offered as help in this regard:

1. The researcher must give first priority to obtaining true and accurate research results, even at the risk of not getting published, tenured, or promoted. If the researcher doubts whether the research is accurate, he or she should seek the advice and counsel of other, more experienced investigators. Multiple heads are always better than one when it comes to detecting subtle flaws or problems in research. The chapter on manuscript writing emphasized the importance of reporting any flaws or problems with the study that the researcher became aware of. The results of the study may still be accurate despite these problems, but the reader of the article needs to be made aware of them so that he or she can properly evaluate the findings.

2. "Controlled" replication of one's own or someone else's research is an excellent means of confirming the truth of research results. Controlled replication means that the study is not replicated exactly as it was originally performed. If an exact replication is performed, the new study may incorporate the same (albeit unknown) fatal flaws that existed in the original study. Controlled replication involves slightly varying certain parameters (e.g., the characteristics of research subjects or the measurement procedures) so that, if the original findings were true, then the new study should obtain similar findings. Of course, the researcher must be aware that some journal editors or some manuscript reviewers may have a negative bias toward publication of replicated studies. They may prefer to publish "totally original and innovative research." This is an unfortunate bias and one that surely has served as one more impediment to the advancement of science.

3. With respect to the published research of other investigators, again, no easy way to determine how accurate their work may be has been identified. In general, however, the more experienced researcher, who has a reputation of doing careful and accurate research and who has numerous publications in well-respected, refereed journals, is more likely to produce accurate research. The new and unknown researcher faces somewhat of an uphill battle in establishing credentials as an honest and thorough investigator. Unfortunately, those researchers who tend to conform to the existing zeitgeist or paradigm, and who publish in the "hot" research areas, face far fewer obstacles in establishing their reputations and in getting their articles accepted for publication. Thus, the human or social nature of the research enterprise again comes into play. Ptolemy was the respected and accepted investigator of his day, while Galileo was the "rogue elephant" who almost got himself burned at the stake!

CHAPTER

9

Finding Monies to Help Pay the Bills

This final chapter considers a number of issues related to obtaining funding for the researcher's project. At many universities and medical centers, limited sources of internal support are available in the form of startup monies or grants to pay expenses of small pilot studies. These grants are likely to be quite small, ranging from a few hundred to a few thousand dollars. They can, however, provide part-time salary monies to hire an assistant (e.g., medical or graduate student, nursing student) to assist in data collection. In many cases, obtaining help with the tedious and time-consuming process of data collection is the single greatest need of the new investigator, whose busy clinical and professional schedule severely restricts the amount of time he or she can devote to the project.

In addition to internal sources of support, a number of external sources also are available that the investigator can approach for support monies. The two basic sources of external funding—private and federal—are described next. Examples of each type and strategies for obtaining funding from the different sources are provided.

Private Foundations

In the United States alone, literally thousands of private foundations or organizations support research in various specialized areas. Many of these groups were established by individual benefactors or families, and their focus can range from a specific problem area to a subject encompassing a wide variety of areas. Examples of family-type foundations are the Joseph P. Kennedy Foundation (for mental retardation research), the Sloan Foundation, and the Donnie and Marie Osmond Foundation (for deafness research). Other private foundations are national associations or organizations, made up of sometimes hundreds or thousands of members, with a focus on specific healthcare problems. Examples of such disorder-based foundations are the National Multiple Sclerosis Society, the American Epilepsy Society, the Deafness Research Foundation, the American Cancer Society, and the American Heart Association. A variety of publications are available as sources of information about specific foundations. Most major libraries and the sponsored research offices at medical centers or medical schools, colleges, and universities all maintain updated collections of "foundation directories" in various specialty areas (education, healthcare, and so on). Some computerized databases (e.g., Sponsored Programs Information Network [SPIN]) also are available that allow the researcher to search for potential funding sources. Some of the foundation directories limit their listings to state or regional foundations or organizations, whereas others are national in scope.

The strategy for obtaining funding from private organizations or foundations involves three steps: (1) search and identify, (2) contact and inquire, and (3) apply and wait. In order to have the greatest chance of obtaining private funding, the researcher should have a project already thoroughly planned and designed. Private foundation people are more impressed by specific and detailed research plans that need funding than they are by what may appear to be preliminary or even vague ideas for possible research studies.

After the researcher has designed the research study, the first step in seeking funding is to search through the appropriate foundation listings and identify those that might possibly fund the project. If at all possible, the researcher should enlist the assistance of other experienced researchers or the staff of sponsored research offices at local medical centers or universities. These people may know of specific foundations that might be likely to fund the researcher's project or, with luck, they might even have personal contacts at a particular foundation and could put in a good word for the researcher. The next step is to write a letter to the contact person designated in the directory listing, or to the foundation director, and make an initial inquiry into the possibility of obtaining funding. The letter should be prepared using a word processor in a neat and professional style (with no typos or grammatical faux pas!) and be no longer than two pages. It should clearly describe, using as little technical jargon as possible, the general goals and objectives of the project, and explain why the project needs to be done and why the researcher needs funding in order to do it. Indicate in the letter that the researcher would appreciate the opportunity to meet with the foundation director (or contact person) to discuss the project in greater detail. Then the researcher will need to wait two weeks and follow up the letter with a phone call (unless, of course, he or she receives a rejection letter or phone call in the meantime).

If the foundation or agency is interested in possibly funding the researcher's project, the researcher may be requested to schedule a personal visit to meet with foundation staff. Thorough preparation for the meeting is essential. A recommended step is for the researcher to write a detailed description of the research project in its entirety, to be read over repeatedly to ensure that he or she is clear on all facets of the project. Armed with this knowledge, the researcher will be able to answer any questions that the foundation people may ask. This document is not to be taken into the meeting, however—the foundation people will not be favorably impressed if they see the researcher looking at notes before answering their questions. The researcher should be knowledgeable and spontaneous, without sounding like a tape recording. The researcher can, however, arrive at the meeting with a detailed written budget request in hand that lists all of the specific equipment, supplies, personnel, and so on, needed for the study, and what each item would cost. No one expects the researcher to remember model numbers and specific prices. Foundation personnel will, however, appreciate the fact that the researcher has gathered this important information.

More frequently, however, the organization or foundation will ask the researcher to submit a formal written proposal for the project. In some cases, they will provide application forms complete with detailed instructions, word or page length limitations, and so on.

In other cases, they may request the submission of a formal written proposal with considerably less specific guidelines regarding how they expect it to be prepared. The writing of the research proposal is similar in many respects to the writing of a publication manuscript. Many excellent published sources are available that describe, in detail, how to go about writing successful grant applications. Consulting one of these sources for use in preparing the application is strongly encouraged. An additional recommendation is for the new investigator to obtain the active assistance of an experienced grant writer in preparing this first application—perhaps a colleague at the researcher's own institution, or someone across town at the local university. The researcher also may consider soliciting the help of someone based at another institution, although this may require exchanging drafts via the mail. Today, this process can be speeded up greatly by using e-mails with file attachments containing parts or all of the written proposal. Whatever route the researcher selects in this regard, it also is highly recommended to allow plenty of time to prepare the application. Waiting until the last minute to start writing is hardly likely to give good results. When it comes to grant writing, haste makes waste, and so does procrastination!

Federal Funding Sources

In the healthcare professions, the single largest source of federal research support is the *National Institutes of Health* (NIH), located in Bethesda, Maryland. As the name indicates, the NIH is composed of at least 20 separate institutes, each devoted to funding projects in specific healthcare areas. Examples are the National Institute on Aging, the National Cancer Institute, the National Institute on Deafness and Other Communication Disorders, the National Institute for Nursing Research, and the National Institute of Mental Health. Each of the different Institutes supports projects with budgets ranging from a few thousand to several million dollars and durations of 1 to 5 or more years (and, frequently, with renewals for additional years). Grants may be awarded to support the training or education of individual scientists (e.g., postdoctoral fellowships), or to support the research projects of individual scientists (e.g., R01s, Research Career Development awards) or groups of scientists (e.g., program project or center grants). The NIH accepts applications with three or four (depending on the nature of the grant) specific deadlines each year. The researcher is provided with a very detailed set of application forms and is expected to comply with a rigid set of guidelines on how to write the grant. The supporting documentation (e.g., budget pages and justification, biographical sketches of the investigators, description of research facilities) frequently is longer than the actual description of the proposed research studies.

Most of the grant applications processed at the NIH are *unsolicited* proposals, in which the investigators apply for funding to support their own original research projects. At times, however, the NIH staff, with advice from professionals in various fields, will identify special needs for new research in specific areas. In such instances, the NIH will issue a special *request for proposals (RFP)* and solicit applications from researchers. The NIH publishes a special document entitled *NIH Guide for Grants and Contracts* that the individual researcher can subscribe to at no cost. It also is possible for the researcher to go directly to the particular NIH institute's website and read or download this document directly. This guide, which is issued four times per year, lists and describes specific RFPs for specific projects, and provides instructions on how to go about applying for these special monies. It is strongly recommended that the researcher either subscribe to this guide or periodically review it (either directly at the institute's website, or at local medical center and university research offices, which will have hard copies available) for possible sources of funding. With these grants, which frequently are more like contracts than grants, the researcher usually will be required to conform to the desires of the NIH, rather than to certain personal ideas about the goals and objectives of the project, but it nevertheless is an excellent way for the researcher to obtain funding for research in his or her specialty area.

When the researcher's grant application arrives at the NIH, it undergoes a complex sequence of processing and review. The first step is the determination of which of the different institutes the grant should go to for review. This determination is made according to the title and content of the application. All NIH grants require the researcher to write a short summary paragraph at the beginning of the application that gives an overview of the project and must contain a number of underlined *keywords* that identify the specific field or subject area of the research. The administrative staff at the NIH will use this information to determine which institute to assign the application for review. If the project involves investigating the effects of certain neural diseases on hearing or language function, for example, the grant will be sent to the National Institute on Deafness and Other Communication Disorders; if the grant is concerned with investigating a possible treatment for cancer, it will be sent to the National Cancer Institute; and so forth. When the grant arrives at the appropriate Institute, it will be assigned to a special *study section* for review.

The study section is made up of a group of 10 to 15 professionals who are appointed to serve on the study section for a period of 3 years. The study section is the essence of the NIH peer review system. Each member theoretically is a "peer" of the grant applicant. These are people who are recognized as established scientists and researchers and who are believed to be the most qualified to judge the scientific soundness and importance of proposals for new research in their respective fields. They have full-time positions as faculty or researchers, typically at a medical school or university. They travel to Bethesda, Maryland, three or four times per year and spend several days locked up in hotel rooms reading and reviewing large stacks of grant applications. At the actual study section meeting, one or more of the members are appointed to be *primary reviewers* of the grant. They are required to thoroughly read and digest the application so that they can lead the group discussion of the relative merits of the proposed project. At the end of the discussion, all members of the study section cast a vote that collectively assigns a rank value to the researcher's proposal.

The ranking of the researcher's proposal relative to all of the other applications reviewed by the study section will determine the probability of funding. From year to year, depending on congressional appropriations, the total amount of money that is allotted to a particular Institute will vary. In awarding grants, the NIH starts with the top-ranked proposal and goes down the list until all of the money is spent. In good years, the probability of the researcher's grant getting funded might be as "good" as 1 in 4; during a bad year, it might be no better than 1 in 10. Thus, the good news is that the NIH funds larger projects over typically longer periods of time, thereby providing the researcher more stability in the planned research activities. The bad news is that, because of the odds being stacked against getting funded, the researcher must devote considerable time and energy in developing the project and preparing the grant application.

The Writing of the Grant Application

As recommended previously, the new investigator, in writing a first grant application, should seek out the assistance and advice of someone who has experience with successful grant writing. (My own mentor in this process was Dr. William D. Neff, a pioneer in the field of auditory neurophysiology.) Although every grant application, like every research project, is unique in many ways, some common rules or guidelines are known to be critical in determining the probability of any particular grant's getting funded.

Some Suggested Do's and Do Not's for Getting Funded

As indicated earlier in this book, at any given moment in the history of science, some topics are "hot" and some are not. "Hot" topics are research areas that a large percentage of the scientific community feels should receive the highest priority for funding. Currently, research on the acquired immunodeficiency syndrome (AIDS) is a good example of a hot area. Other topics are not "hot" simply because a majority of scientists feel that the research area has already been adequately investigated or that little relevant or important new information is likely to develop from research in that area. The majority opinion (prevailing zeitgeist), however, is not always accurate. (Recall, from a previous chapter, the consequences of Galileo's challenge to Ptolemy's view that the earth is the center of the universe!) Even though the researcher may sincerely believe that he or she is correct, it must be remembered that those who advocate the "minority opinion" may have difficulty getting funded. It is of little comfort to know that people like Galileo would, in today's peer review system, probably have had his grant rejected also. Therefore, the prudent choice of a research topic frequently is one that does conform to the prevailing zeitgeist.

An insightful and very useful classification of the "fundability" of potential research studies was proposed by Dr. Bert O'Malley, a colleague at Baylor College of Medicine in the mid-1970s. O'Malley, an extremely competent and experienced cell biologist, suggested that, in terms of the probability of getting funding, research studies can be rank-ordered in three levels, starting with studies that have the highest likelihood of being funded and proceeding to those that are least likely to be funded. The three levels are characterized as follows:

- *Highest level*: NEW questions that will be answered using NEW research tools or technology

- *Middle level*: OLD questions that will be answered using NEW technology, or NEW questions that will be answered using OLD technology

- *Lowest level*: OLD questions that will be answered using OLD tools or OLD technology

As suggested by this ranking, from the viewpoint of the peer reviewers, new questions usually are considered more important than old questions, and using the latest scientific tools or technology usually is better than using older technologies. Experienced authors (such as myself) who recognize the truth of this assessment unfortunately may not always heed its wisdom; nevertheless, the new researcher is urged to take this ranking concept into serious consideration when selecting a first research topic area.

The chances of obtaining external funding improve astronomically if the new investigator can gather some research data that demonstrate the importance of the proposed study. This important process is referred to as *obtaining pilot data*. A *pilot study* can be defined as a preliminary investigation that provides research data to support the feasibility and importance of the researcher's proposed project. With new PhDs, this may be the doctoral dissertation research project. If the dissertation project has already been published and is now "ancient history," the researcher will need to conduct new research for use in supporting the grant application. It is almost a universal law that, without solid and convincing supporting research, research grant applications to the NIH are almost certain to be rejected. The study section members must be convinced that the research idea is not only important but also feasible and that the researcher has the skills and experience to successfully carry the project through to a successful conclusion. A track record of earlier successful research in the particular topic area, or newly generated pilot data, is what the reviewers will want to see.

Second, it goes almost without saying that the grant proposal must be presented in a neat, attractive, and professional manner.

The researcher is trying to sell a product to a group of skeptical and sometimes grumpy study section reviewers. The study section members may be grumpy simply because they have been locked away in a hotel room for hours at a time, reading an endless supply of different applications. The researcher should keep this fact in mind when writing the application. Some tips for accomplishing this follow:

- Make the reading as easy as possible.

- Use frequent paragraph breaks.

- Clearly separate important sections with well-worded and concise headings.

- Summarize important information frequently.

- Underline important words, concepts, or phrases.

Although the primary reviewers must read and digest every word of the proposal, the other reviewers may, on occasion, only skim the proposal, rather than reading it in detail. The writing should ensure that even those readers who skim the document will still be sold on the importance and feasibility of the project.

Also, a bit of politicking is in order! The researcher should visit the Institute's website or go to the research office of the medical center or local university to find out who is currently serving on the study section that may review the submitted grant application. NIH publishes this information for public knowledge. The names of the study section members should then be researched to determine if any of them have published in the researcher's particular topic area; if this is the case, the researcher should be sure to read their articles and cite them (favorably, if at all possible, of course) in the application. If a study section member is recognized as having a strong negative bias toward the researcher's area of study, the researcher may wish to request that the grant be reviewed at another study section, or wait until that person leaves the study section before submitting the application.

And, finally, but perhaps most important, the budding researcher must not give up the idea of the proposed project if the grant application is rejected. Whether the grant is funded or not, the researcher will receive a detailed written critique of the proposal. This document summarizes the study section members' views regarding the major strengths and weaknesses of the proposed research. Even with grants that are awarded, this critique may still provide the researcher with useful suggestions on how the project can be improved or strengthened. If, however, the grant is not funded, this critique can serve as an extremely valuable guide for redesigning the research study or rewriting the grant application for resubmission. In rewriting the grant application, the researcher must clearly spell out in the new application what changes have been made in response to the reviewers' critique, and where in the application these changes can be found. The revised application is then resubmitted to the Institute and will go to the same study section for a second review. If the changes made by the researcher are acceptable to the reviewers, the grant probably will receive a relatively higher rank score than it did in the initial review. With luck, the new rank score may be high enough to bring the application into the fundable range for the new collection of grant applications being reviewed by the study section. If the original application contained pilot or supporting research data, it would be well worth the researcher's time and effort to collect additional supporting data, if possible, to include with the revised application. The study section members probably will be favorably impressed by this demonstration of the researcher's tenacity and perseverance!

Once again, a multitude of excellent published guides on how to write grant applications are available. A good way to start this search, however, is with the comprehensive book on this subject by Hall (1988).

References and
Suggested Readings

Bach-Y-Rita, P. (1990). Brain plasticity as a basis for recovery of function in humans. *Neuropsychologia, 12,* 547–554.

Bishop, B. (1982). Neural plasticity. *Physical Therapy, 62,* 1122–1143.

Barber, T. X. (1976). *Pitfalls in human research.* New York: Pergamon Press.

Cohen, J. (1977). *Statistical power analysis for the behavioral sciences.* New York: Academic Press.

Cohen, J. (1988). *Statistical power analysis for the behavioral sciences* (2nd ed.). Mihwah, NH: Lawrence Erlbaum Associates.

Cotman, C. W. (1985). *Synaptic plasticity.* New York: Guilford Press.

Cureton, E. E., & D'Agostino, R. B. (1983). *Factor analysis: An applied approach.* Hillsdale, NJ: Lawrence Erlbaum Associates.

Gorsuch, R. L. (1983). *Factor analysis* (2nd ed.). Hillsdale, NJ: Lawrence Erlbaum Associates.

Hall, M. (1988). *Getting funded: A complete guide to proposal writing.* Portland, OR: Continuing Education Publications.

Hegde, M. N. (1993). *Clinical research in communicative disorders: Principles and strategies* (2nd. ed). Austin, TX: Pro-Ed.

Johnson, W. (1955). A study of the onset and development of stuttering. In W. Johnson & R. R. Lautenegger (Eds.), *Stuttering in children and adults* (pp. 37–73). Minneapolis: University of Minnesota Press.

Johnson, W., & Associates. (1959). *The onset of stuttering.* Minneapolis: University of Minnesota Press.

Kearns, K. P. (1986). Flexibility of single-subject experimental designs. Part III: Design selection and arrangement of experimental phases. *Journal of Speech and Hearing Disorders, 51,* 204–214.

Keppel, G. (1991). *Design and analysis: A researcher's handbook.* Upper Saddle River, NJ: Prentice Hall.

Kerren, G., & Lewis, C. (1979). Partial omega squared for ANOVA designs. *Educational and Psychological Measurement, 39,* 119–128.

Kuhn, T. S. (1962). *The structure of scientific revolutions.* Chicago: University of Chicago Press.

Luria, A. R. (1966). *Higher cortical functions in man.* New York: Basic Books [see Chapter 1].

Monge, P. R., & Cappella, J. N. (1980). *Multivariate techniques in human communication research.* New York: Academic Press.

McReynolds, L. V., & Kearns, K. P. (1983). *Single-subject experimental designs in communicative disorders.* Baltimore: University Park Press.

McReynolds, L. V., & Kearns, K. P. (1986). Flexibility of single-subject experimental designs. Part I: A review of the basics of single-subject designs. *Journal of Speech and Hearing Disorders, 51*, 194–203.

Pedhazur, E. J. (1999). *Multiple regression in behavioral research* (3rd ed.). New York: Harcourt Brace.

Roberts, J, Wallace, I., & Henderson, F. (Eds.). (1997). *Otitis media in young children: Medical, developmental, and educational consequences.* Baltimore: Paul H. Brookes.

Runyon, R., Haber, A., & Reese, P. (1976). *Fundamentals of behavioral statistics* (3rd ed.). Reading, MA: Addison-Wesley.

Schiavetti, N., & Metz, D. E. (2002). *Evaluating research in communicative disorders* (4th ed.). Boston: Allyn & Bacon.

Siegel, S. (1956). *Nonparametric statistics in the behavioral sciences.* New York: McGraw-Hill.

Siegel, S. (1988). *Nonparametric statistics for the behavioral sciences* (2nd ed.). New York: McGraw-Hill.

Steel, R. G. D., Torrie, J. H., & Dickey, D. A. (1997). *Principles and procedures of statistics.* New York: McGraw-Hill.

The American Heritage College Dictionary. (2000). Boston: Houghton Mifflin Company.

Weiss-Lambrou, R. (1989). *The health professionals guide to writing for publication.* Springfield, IL: Charles C Thomas.

Winer, B. J. (1991). *Statistical principles in experimental design.* New York: McGraw-Hill.

Index

Note: page number in bold reference non-text material.